The" Indigenous American Herbal Bible: 6 in
1 Book of Ancestral Medicinal Plants with
images"

By

Joseph F . Peraza

The" Indigenous American Herbal Bible: 6 in 1 Book of Ancestral Medicinal Plants with images".

Introduction: Table of contents

HERBAL BIBLE BOOK 1

Chapter 1 Native American Medicine

Introduction:Table of Contents

CHAPTER 1
2.1 Herb Preservation
2.2 Making Salves
2.3 Poultice
2.4 Smudging

HERBAL BIBLE BOOK 3

Introduction: Table of contents

CHAPTER 1: THE WHEEL
1.1 Glossary of Native American Tradition
1.2 The Native American Medicine Wheel
1.3 The Sacred Pipe Ceremony
1.4 Sweat Lodge

CHAPTER 2:NATIVE AMERICAN HERBS.

2.1 Horsetail
2.2 Lemon Balm
2.3 Nettle
2.4 Ginseng
2.5 Wild Ginger

HERBAL BIBLE BOOK 4

Introduction: Table of contents

CHAPTER 1: Herbs In Native American

CHAPTER 2

HERBAL BIBLE BOOK 5

Introduction: Table of content

CHAPTER 1: HOME MADE HERBAL SOLUTIONS FOR DISEASES

1.1 Asthma and it's Herbal Remedies

1.2 Backache and it's Herbal Remedies

1.3 Allergies,rashes and it's herbal remedies

1.4 Sore throat and it's Herbal Remedies

CHAPTER 2

2.1 Cramps and it's Herbal Remedies

2.2 Acne and it's Herbal Remedies

2.3 Anemia and it's Herbal Remedies

2.4 Stress and it's Herbal Remedies

HERBAL BIBLE BOOK 6

Introduction: Table of content

CHAPTER 1:

1.1 Fibroid and it's Herbal Remedies

1.2 Cold,Cough and it's Herbal Remedies

INTRODUCTION

The" Indigenous American Herbal Bible: 6 in 1 Book of Ancestral Medicinal Plants with images" is a knowledge compendium that immerses compendiums in the rich realm of Native American herbalism, furnishing a comprehensive and illuminating disquisition of indigenous traditions and healing practices.

This fascinating book, in five unique volumes, attests to the abecedarian relationship between Native American societies and the natural terrain.

The first portion of this expansive study exposes compendiums to the cornucopia of medicinal sauces that have played an important part in Native American societies' mending practices for decades. It reveals the mending powers and spiritual significance of shops similar to savant, cedar, and sweetgrass.

The alternate book dives into the spiritual side of Native American herbalism, shining light on the holy solemnities and observances that shops use to bring mending, protection, and connection to the godly. It emphasizes the deep conviction in the interdependence of all life forms, as well as the reverence for Mother Earth and her immolations.

The final member invites callers to probe the ancient remedial procedures used by Native American herbalists. From plasters and teas to smudging and energy cleaning, these time- recognized practices offer vital perceptivity into indigenous communities' holistic approach to health and well- being.

The fourth volume provides a unique perspective on Native American ecological understanding. It demonstrates their environmentally conscious harvesting practices and great regard for the natural world, emphasizing the significance of balance and harmony in all relations with the natural world.

The book's last section weaves all of these aspects together into a shade of wisdom that celebrates the complicated web of life and the function of sauces within it. It's a resource for anyone interested in incorporating Native American herbalism into their lives, furnishing practical advice as well as a deeper knowledge of the artistic and spiritual significance of these practices.

The" Indigenous American Herbal Bible: 6 in 1 Book of Ancestral Medicinal Plants with images" is a knowledge treasure trove that takes compendiums on a transubstantiation trip into the core of indigenous traditions.

This book is an engaging and instructional resource for anybody interested in herbal drugs, indispensable drugs, or the profound wisdom of Native American traditions. It emphasizes the significance of conserving and honoring traditional traditions that have supported communities for glories while also furnishing significant perceptivity into nature's mending capability.

HERBAL BIBLE BOOK 1

CHAPTER 1

1.1 NATIVE AMERICAN MEDICINE

Native American medicine is based on healthy living beliefs,the outcomes of disease and sickness producing habits , and the spiritual principles that help restore the Balance Almost all tribes have these same beliefs but nevertheless, the techniques of diagnosis and treatment differ widely from tribe to tribe and healer to healer.

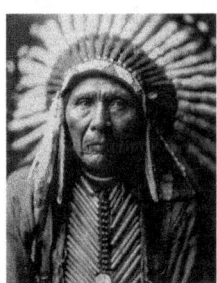**Native American Dress**

Origins

Native American healing techniques have been practiced in North America for at least 12,000 years, and potentially as long as 40,000 years. Although the phrase Native American medicine implies a standardized healing system, there are around 500 indigenous peoples in North America, each reflecting a diverse wealth of healing knowledge, rituals, and ceremonies.

Many components of Native American healing are kept hidden and have not been documented. The traditions are passed down orally through elders, through vision quests, and through initiation. It is considered that imparting therapeutic knowledge too openly or casually can undermine the medicine's spiritual effectiveness.

Many Native American healers, on the other hand, recognise that writing down their healing practices is a method to conserve these traditions for future generations. Many people feel that sharing their healing practices and values will help everyone achieve a healthy balance with nature and all forms of life.

Benefits

Anyone who really aspires to live a life of fullness and balance can benefit from Native American medicine. These advantages could be physical, emotional, or spiritual. There is an understanding, however, that "the diseases of civilization," or white man's maladies, frequently require white man's medication. In such circumstances,

Native American medicine can be an important component of a holistic healing strategy. The most successful programmes in Native communities, for example, have integrated Western approaches to psychological counseling, social work, and traditional Native American healing practices.

Inherited problems such as birth abnormalities or retardation are difficult to treat using Native American medicine. Native healers also think that some ailments are caused by a patient's actions. They will sometimes refuse to treat a patient because they do not want to interfere with the patient's need to acquire life lessons.

Other ailments are not treated because they are considered "callings" or "initiation diseases." Medicine is defined by some Native healers as "the calling that comes in the form of a dream or life experiences

Description

Native American medicine is founded on a spiritual understanding of existence. A healthy individual is someone who has a feeling of purpose and follows the Great Spirit's guidance. Every person has this counsel written on their heart.

A person must be committed to a path of beauty, harmony, and balance in order to be healthy. Gratitude, respect, and generosity are also seen to be necessary for living a healthy life. "Health means the restoration of the body, mind, and spirit to balance the wholeness of life energy in the body," explains Ken Cohen.

sickness cause theories and even sickness nomenclature differ from tribe to tribe. Diseases are assumed to have either internal or external causes, or both. The most important internal cause of sickness is negative thinking.

Negative thinking encompasses sentiments of shame, blame, low self-esteem, avarice, despair, worry, melancholy, wrath, jealousy, and self-centeredness, among other things.You Can do yourself more harm than any other evil sorcerer if care is not taken Diseases can also have extrinsic causes.

A person is more vulnerable to hazardous germs if their life is unbalanced, they have a weak constitution, they indulge in negative thinking, or they are under a lot of stress. Other persons or spirits could also be at blame for an illness. Environmental toxins are another external source of sickness. These toxins include alcohol, contaminated air, water, and some foods.

Native American healers believe that physical, emotional, or spiritual trauma can also cause disease. These traumas can cause mental and emotional pain, soul loss, and spiritual power loss. In these circumstances, the healer must employ ritual and other means to physically return the patient's soul and power. Some diseases are caused by people breaking the "rules for living." Respect for animals, people, locations, ritual objects, events, or spirits may be included in these rules.

Native American healers use a variety of approaches to diagnose illnesses. A discussion of one's symptoms, personal and family history, examination of nonverbal signs such as posture or tone of voice, and medical divination are examples of these. The healer's intuition, sensitivity, and spiritual strength are more significant than the specific technique.

There is no such thing as a normal Native American healing session. Prayer, chanting, music, smudging (burning sage or aromatic woods), herbs, laying-on of hands, massage, counseling, imagery, fasting, harmonizing with nature, dreaming, sweat lodges, taking hallucinogens (e.g., peyote), developing inner silence, going on a shamanic journey, and ceremony are all methods of healing. Many healing sessions include family and community members.

Healing can occur swiftly at times. Sometimes considerable time is required for healing. The intensity of the therapy is thought to be more crucial than the time necessary. Even if the recovery occurs rapidly, a change in lifestyle is frequently required to make the healing last.

In Native American healing, a medicine bundle can also be employed. The medicine bundle is a leather or animal fur pouch in which the healer keeps ritual objects, charms, herbs, stones, and other healing gear. The bundle is a tangible representation of the medicine power bestowed to the healer by the spirits, either for general healing or for the treatment of a specific sickness. Bundles differ according to clan, tribe, and individual.

Unless the practitioner is a licensed health care provider, Native American medicine is not covered by insurance. The majority of Native healers do not have a defined cost for their services. Healing is seen as "a gift from the Great Spirit." However, gifts for the healer are welcomed.

Offering a gift "ensures treatment success because healing spirits appreciate generosity." Groceries, clothing, money, or another personal expression of respect and appreciation may be given as gifts.

Often, the only present required is a pouch of tobacco.

Preparations

The medicine person informs the patient about the necessary preparations for the healing ceremony.

Precautions

A medicine person is required to ensure safe Native American medicine healing. People with hypertension should keep an eye on their blood pressure during a sweat lodge ceremony. When sage or cedar is used in a ceremony, people who have asthma may have problems. People who are claustrophobic may find the sweat lodge's intimate, hot, and dark setting unbearable.

Adverse Effects

Some herbs can produce nausea, vomiting, or diarrhea. These reactions are frequently welcomed by Native Americans and seen as a type of purging or cleansing of the physical body.

General Acceptance & Research

Native American healing practices have received no formal scientific research. Medicine practitioners do not write down their practises for fear of them being misappropriated by others who are not schooled in their sacred ways. Native Americans and anyone seeking a spiritually based approach to medicine are the most prominent users of this style of medicine.

Certification And Training

For thousands of years, Native American medicine has been passed down through word of mouth. Healing power can be inherited from ancestors, received from another healer, or gained via training and initiation.

Healers often receive their training from a single primary tutor. With the accessibility of long-distance travel and communication, many healers now have multiple mentors. Training to be a healer is a lengthy process that needs strength, sacrifice, and patience.

1.2 A BRIEF OVERVIEW OF NATIVE AMERICAN MEDICINE.

The majority of the Native Americans descended entirely from a single group of migrants that crossed over the Bering land bridge between Asia and America that existed more than 15,000 years ago.

They adopted a hunter-gatherer society – men would hunt for large animals while the women would forage for fruits and any other edible plant-based food and hunt for small animals. Everything was shared with the whole tribe so they did not waste food as they couldn't store any surplus.

When a large animal, such as a bison (Bison bison), was killed, that entire animal was used, there was no refrigeration, so the meat was distributed amongst everyone, cooked to eat directly or smoked to make jerky for eating later. The bones and teeth were used to make weapons, personal decoration and fishhooks, and the skin was used for clothing, shoes or patching up tepees.

The origins of Native American healing practice and ceremony are as diverse and rich as the tribes themselves.

And the healing practices varied widely from tribe to tribe, involving various rituals, ceremonies, and a diverse wealth of healing knowledge.

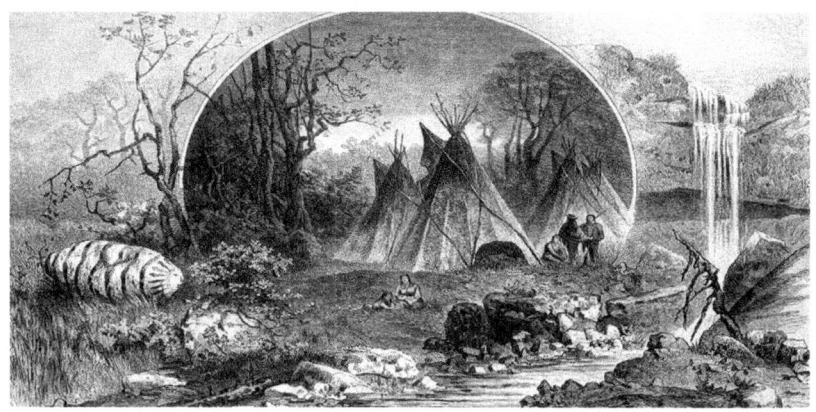

At the heart of this would be the tribes' medicine man who was the spiritual guide of the tribe and its leader in an emergency, often holding a position equivalent to that of the war chief.

Most tribes believed that health was an expression of the spirit and a continual process of staying strong spiritually, mentally, and physically. Each person was responsible for their own health, and all thoughts and actions had consequences, including illness, disability, bad luck, or trauma.

There had to be balance and harmony between themselves, those around them and their natural environment. If this was correct, "the Creator" would keep them away from illness or harm and health could be restored. Not surprisingly, herbal remedies filled an essential role within these healing practices, stretching beyond the body's aches and pains and into the realm of spirituality and harmony.

In 1832, George Catlin, the American adventurer, lawyer, painter, author, and traveller spent some time with the Mandan tribe who lived on the Knife River in Dakota. While there he met Old Bear, the tribe's medicine man and watched as he instructed new students in the ceremonial practices of the tribe and showed them the collection and use of herbal remedies.

Although most herbs and natural products were gathered from their surrounding environment it has been theorized that if certain items were unavailable they would be traded for often over long distances.

Tobacco And Cedar

The Creator gave Native Americans the Four Sacred Medicines to be used in everyday life and ceremonies; they are tobacco, sage, cedar and sweetgrass. All of them can be used to smudge (burning herbs and plants to release an aromatic smoke), though sage, cedar and sweetgrass also have many other uses. The tribal elders would say that the spirits liked the aroma produced when the sacred medicines were burned.

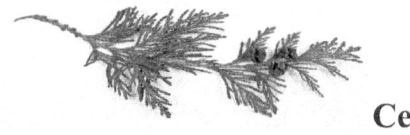

Cedar

Indian Tobacco (Lobelia inflata) has a long-standing cultural history among native people, recognised as the first gift the creator bestowed upon the native people. The herbaceous plants are annual or biennial, growing up to 100 cm tall, with tiny hairs covering the stems.

The burning of tobacco during ceremonies honored and welcomed guests in the sharing of a sacred peace pipe, but it also blessed food crops and an upcoming hunt, provided communication with the Creator, and bound agreements between tribes to ensure the general welfare of the community.

The tobacco plant was used by the Cherokee, Iroquois, Penobscot, and other indigenous peoples as a poultice or cold infusion to heal body aches, bites and stings, abscesses, or sores. It was chewed, made into an infusion, or a tincture for its emetic properties (it is often referred to as "puke weed") and to help with a sore throat, asthma, or the prevention of colic.

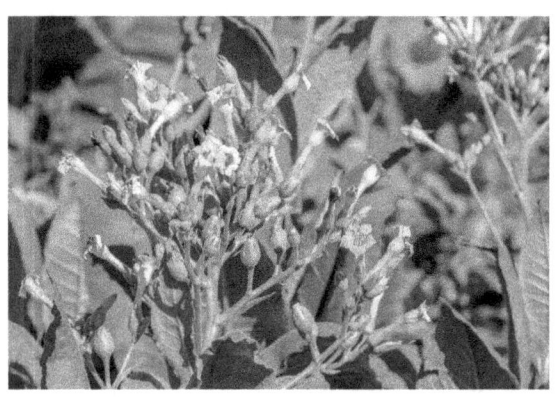

Tobacco leaf

The Iroquois used the roots to treat venereal diseases and the Cherokee burned the foliage to smoke out gnats and unwelcome insects. However, consuming lobelia, especially the roots, can cause some extreme adverse effects, including sweating, diarrhea, tremors, rapid heartbeat, mental confusion, convulsions, hypothermia, coma, and even death.

If you can imagine cedar trees (Juniperus virginiana) are found in cool, wet forests where fungi and moulds thrive it is not surprising that cedar oils have antioxidant and antibiotic properties which can repel insects, moulds, fungi, bacteria and viruses. Cedar is often used in smudging for purification.

Western Red Cedar leaves have long been a popular internal and external medicine for painful joints among Coastal Native Peoples and are a useful antifungal for skin and nail fungus. It has restorative uses as cedar tea for fighting infections and fevers or as a cough medicine. Some studies indicate that cedar promotes immune function by helping the white blood cells to work better, stimulating the immune cells to fight infection.

Sage and sweetgrass

Sweetgrass (Hierochloe odorata) is a perennial plant with a vanilla-scented aroma that grows in North America, Asia and Europe. It contains coumarin (C9H6O2), which has blood-thinning properties.

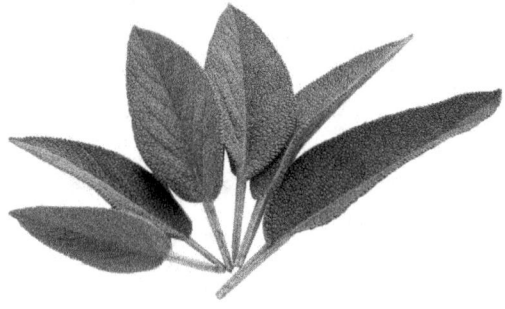

Sage leaf

The Native Americans used it as a purifying herb and as incense in smudging. It is said that the sweet-smelling smoke cleanses the spirit and brings sacred messages to the higher planes of existence. Herbal tea made from the leaves was used to treat coughs, sore throats and fever.

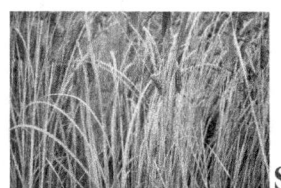 **Sweet Grass**

Sweetgrass Contains Coumarin (C9h6o2) Which Has Blood-thinning Properties

Apart from being mixed with onion to make a tasty accompaniment to the Sunday roast, sage has been used medicinally for generations. Sage (Salvia officinalis) is a perennial, evergreen shrub, with woody stems and grayish leaves.It is native to southern Europe and the Mediterranean region but has been naturalized to other warmer temperate climates, including North America.

Traditionally, sage has been used in attempts to relieve pain, protect against oxidative stress, free radical damage, angiogenesis, inflammation, bacterial and virus infection. Sage is applied directly to the skin for cold sores, gum disease, sore mouth, throat and tongue and swollen, painful nasal passages.

The leaves have been made into poultices and used externally to treat sprains, swelling, ulcers and bleeding. It can be used for digestive problems and women have used sage for painful menstrual periods, to correct excessive milk flow during nursing, and to reduce hot flushes.

It was also commonly used in tea form to treat sores and it is also considered one of the good herbs for coughs. Some studies have claimed that essential oils of sage can inhibit the enzyme acetylcholinesterase (AChE), which is responsible for degrading and inactivating acetylcholine in Alzheimer's disease.

Well-tried efficacy

The American missionary John Heckewelder (1743–1823) noted that in Native American tribes there were physicians of both sexes, who would take considerable pains to acquire a correct knowledge of the properties and medical virtues of plants, roots and barks, for the benefit of their patients. And that their science was founded on observation, experience and the well-tried efficacy of the remedies being used.

Frances Densmore (1867–1957) the American anthropologist and ethnographer observed during her travels that the practitioners were able to heal wounds and cure diseases by the simple application of natural herbal remedies. She also noted that different healers often knew individual medicinal plants by multiple names, some unique to a particular individual, and would gather and collect the herbs at the proper seasons, sometimes fetching them from the distance of several days' journey from their homes, then they would cure or dry them properly, tie them up in small bundles, and preserve them for later use.

Conclusions

Some of the Native American tribes have become immortalized through numerous reruns of old western films; the Apaches, the Cherokee or the Sioux and their chiefs live on in history – Sitting Bull, Geronimo and Crazy Horse. In reality, it was a history of greed, tragedy and betrayal by the colonizing Europeans. What started out as the mutual trade between the indigenous population and the colonists deteriorated over time as imported diseases like smallpox, tuberculosis, measles, cholera, and the bubonic plague decimated the native populations.

The colonists viewed the indigenous people as subordinate and uncivilized due to their nomadic lifestyles and "underutilisation" of the land. Relations worsened and over a period of 300 years, from 1609 to 1900, there were bloody conflicts and involuntary relocation until Native American tribes went from inhabiting their ancestral lands, which could encompass an entire land area, to living on specifically defined native reservations.

Today, many tribes in the United States are now reviving their traditions and cultures from teaching their language to the next generation, holding inter-tribal gatherings and exploring the role of traditional medicine. Native American traditional healing takes the holistic approach on the whole person with herbal remedies, ceremonies, prayers, and the inclusion of the family all being part of the healing journey and today traditional healers have found that combining modern medicine with traditional healing produces better health outcomes than from modern medicine alone.

Native Americans are being encouraged to return to more traditional forms of eating as part of the effort to address health issues like diabetes, obesity and heart disease often associated with a highly processed western diet. Because of this there has been an increasing demand for buffalo meat following studies that have shown the meat to be a leaner and less atherogenic risk than beef.

The buffalo is well-adapted to the wide grass plains as its natural habitat and as a result the meat contains a lower total fat content and provides a more favorable fatty acid composition compared to animals that have spent a greater portion of their life eating corn.

So, there has been a return of the buffalo, nearly hunted to extinction in the 1800s, with many animals now being bred for commercial purposes on farms and herds reintroduced into national parks as a part of conservation breeding programmes. Bison are migratory herbivores who move across large areas, grazing almost exclusively on grasses, the result being that other plants normally dominated or overshadowed grow better, creating a more diverse mosaic of habitats.

The bison also modify the environment by trampling woody vegetation, wallowing (rolling on the ground repeatedly to avoid biting insects and to shed loose fur), digesting vegetation and excreting their waste across large areas, which increases seed dispersal and nutrients over the landscape. This behavior helps to increase arthropod, amphibian and plant diversity.

This biodiversity has seen the increase of birds such as the greater prairie chicken or the scaled and bobwhite quails. Larger animals like the pronghorn antelope and mule deer are among the large mammals that benefit as the bison grazing increases the abundance of forbs (herbaceous flowering plants) and shrubs that constitute the dietary mainstays of both species.

Just as the reintroduction of gray wolves into Yellowstone national park had a positive effect on the park ecosystem, perhaps the return of the buffalo will help to rewild the great plains for the benefit of everyone.

1.3 BENEFITS OF HERBAL MEDICINE

Herbal therapy has long been recognised as a reliable technique of healing for over 60,000 years at least and this is based on archaeological findings. According to the World Health Organisation, three-quarters of the world's population now uses herbs for basic healthcare.

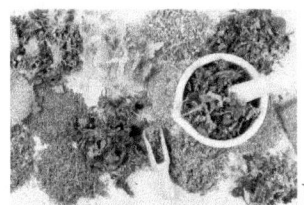
Herbs

MeanWhile it falls under the umbrella of complementary medicine, it is inextricably linked to achieving optimal general wellbeing, healing, and holistic preventative action. When utilized correctly, the knock-on effect of these benefits can be life-changing.The listed bellow are the primary advantages of practicing the use of herbal medication Low-cost and easily accessible

Herbs of high quality should always be taken in controlled doses as directed by a certified naturopath. This step in the process of obtaining herbs is sometimes perceived as an expensive one, however this is (according to recognised naturopaths) a bit of a fallacy.

With most general practitioners no longer offering bulk billing, seeing a naturopath for herbal medicine is a more cost-effective choice. The correct herbs can help with disease prevention, overall health and well-being, and treatment of disorders. Herbs can have extraordinarily high efficacy in relatively modest amounts when used alone or in conjunction with pharmaceuticals (which must always be disclosed to your naturopath). So, for a relatively low price, a little goes a long way. Effective herbs will also reduce your visits to your naturopath and general practitioner.

Natural treatment

Herbs are a completely natural method to health prevention, treatment, and maintenance. When used correctly and especially tailored for your needs, they are a safe and effective way of avoiding or supplementing pharmaceutical medications in some cases.When properly used,there are few drawbacks to include herbal medicines into your overall health routine.
Side effect risk has been reduced.

Unlike many prescription treatments, herbal medicine has considerably fewer negative effects when used as directed.Their composition is purely to maintain and strengthen the body continuously . Despite their tremendous efficacy, they have far fewer cases of adverse reactions, reliance, and problems. If you decide to quit using herbal medicine, you will not experience debilitating withdrawal symptoms (at worst, you may have a recurrence of the symptoms you were hoping to eliminate with the herbs, but at a lower intensity).

You Can Safely Experiment With Various Herbs.

High quality natural medicinal herbs can be trialed and evaluated in a safe manner with little downtime as long as they are under the supervision of a professional. While we may ask you to wait a particular length of time between trying herbs, this is usually done to allow us to properly measure how and if it is working for you.

1.4 NATIVE HERBS HEALING PROPERTIES

Native Americans have utilized whole plants for millennia to treat disease, and while they knew the medicines helped, they didn't always know why. Teas made from pine needles or rose hips, for example, were used to treat colds and flu. The vitamin C and bioflavonoids in pine needles and rose hips, as we now know, were responsible for the therapeutic action.

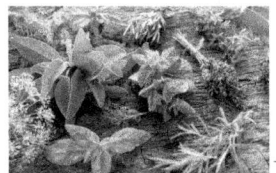 **Herbs**

Science is now recognising the medicinal properties of herbs, such as vitamins, minerals, enzymes, and phytochemicals.

•**Glycyrrhizinate:** Glycyrrhizinate are antiviral, anti-inflammatory, and skin-protective phytochemicals found in licorice. They also prevent tumor formation.

•**Alkaloids :** Are found in a variety of plants, including goldenseal. They prevent yeast overgrowth in the body, maintain healthy levels of bacteria in the gastrointestinal and urinary tracts, and help the immune system function.

•**Eleutherosides :** Are compounds found in Siberian ginseng. They improve endurance, stimulate appetite, and boost physical and mental vigor. They activate the metabolism, immunological system, and central nervous system.

Eleutherosides can also help with some of the symptoms of menopause, including irregular periods and hot flashes.

•**Chlorophyll:** All green herbs contain chlorophyll. It combats bacteria, aids in the healing of burns and wounds, and is anti-cancer.Its also popularly known as a rich source of vitamin K

•**Diterpenes:** Diterpenes can be found in a variety of plants, including rosemary. It is an effective antioxidant, anticancer, and anti-liver-toxin agent.

•**Fatty acids:** Essential fatty acids, specifically omega-3 and omega-6 fatty acids, are fats that the body cannot produce. They keep cell membranes and myelin sheaths (the protective covering of nerve fibers) intact. They increase the production of prostaglandins (hormone-like molecules that, among other things, mediate metabolism, smooth muscle activity, and nerve transmission), lower blood cholesterol levels, and boost immunity. They can be found in a variety of plants, including saw palmetto.

•Anthocyanidins: Bilberries, black currants, and raspberries contain anthocyanins, a type of phytochemical.

They combat free radicals (byproducts of metabolic reactions in the body that can lead to degenerative illnesses such as cardiovascular disease and cancer); they reduce blood-vessel plaque formation, thereby maintaining blood flow and lowering the risk of cardiovascular disease; they inhibit edema (swelling caused by fluid accumulation); they fight inflammation; and they improve vision.

•Ginkgolic Acid: Ginkolic acid is another antioxidant present in Ginkgo biloba. It boosts circulation and mental clarity, alleviates depression, and combats cancer.

•Hesperidin: Hesperidin is an antioxidant found in milk thistle seeds that protects capillaries and strengthens cell membranes. It is effective against liver illness and protects against UV rays.

•Isothiocyanates: Horseradish contains isothiocyanates. They stimulate the creation of defensive enzymes and prevent DNA damage, lowering the risk of breast cancer.

•**Gingerols:** Gingerols are antioxidants that aid in protein and fat digestion. They also relieve stomach discomfort and battle liver damage and inflammation. They are the active ingredients in ginger.

•**Phthalides:** Found in parsley, phthalides detoxify carcinogens and increase the synthesis of helpful enzymes.

•**Hypericin:** The active ingredient in St. John's wort is hypericin. It may assist to boost mood by modulating neurotransmitters in the brain.

•**Proanthocyanidins:** Proanthocyanidins are antioxidants present in elderberry and bilberry. They offer protection against cancer, high blood cholesterol, and the influenza virus. They also help to strengthen the walls of blood vessels.

•**Phytochemicals:** Phytochemicals are naturally occurring substances found in plants (the word "phyto" means "plant" in Greek). Herbs and other plants can be used to separate and concentrate these plant components.Some phytochemicals are efficient cancer fighters or antioxidants, while others lower cholesterol, reduce artery plaque, promote immune system activity, or stimulate enzyme production. The phytochemicals listed below are found in many of the herbs used by American Indians over the millennia.

•**Quercetin:** Quercetin is a flavonoid found throughout the plant kingdom.
(Flavonoids are antioxidants that occur naturally in many fruits, vegetables, and other plants.) Quercetin is antihistamine, anti-inflammatory, and anti-cancer. It also helps to stabilize cell membranes and decreases capillary fragility.

•**Phenolic Acids:** Phenolic acids are antioxidants that prevent nitrosamines (cancer-causing chemicals) from forming. Berries, parsley, and all flowering plants contain them.

•**Lipoic Acid:** Found in many plant foods, lipoic acid is a powerful antioxidant that detoxifies the body of heavy metals, protects against cancer and heart disease, normalizes blood sugar levels, and slows aging. Lipoic acid is an important component of energy synthesis.

•**Flavonglycosides:** Flavonglycosides are powerful antioxidants (free radical fighters). They also widen blood vessels, boosting blood flow, increase mental clarity, eyesight and hearing, and aid in the treatment of depression. Ginkgo biloba contains them.

•**Polyacetylenes:** Polyacetylenes are found in parsley as well. They regulate prostaglandin production and protect against carcinogens.

•**Lactones:** Lactones, which are contained in kava kava root, protect the body from cancer by removing carcinogens.

Indigenous herbs have exceptional medical properties that are strongly established in traditional knowledge. These botanical jewels have numerous medicinal benefits, including pain alleviation, immune system fortification, and general wellbeing enhancement. These natural treatments, derived from millennia of expertise, not only treat bodily problems but also improve mental and spiritual well-being.

Native herbs, which embrace a holistic approach to health, represent the tremendous synergy between nature and human well-being, making them a useful resource for people seeking alternative and sustainable paths to recovery.

CHAPTER 2:

2.1 NATIVE AMERICAN HEALING

RITUALS

Since antiquity, healing rituals have been a feature of every religion and belief system. Self-preservation is a powerful instinct that, when joined with true magic, may produce miraculous results. As a result, most traditions contain great therapeutic secrets.

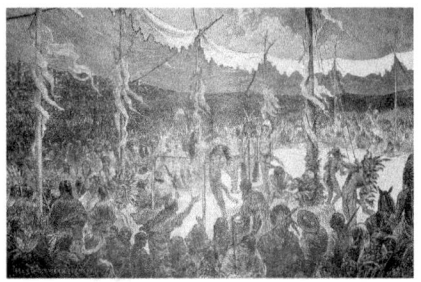

Native Americans

Native American healing practices are thought to be among the most potent. Most likely because they are bold and true.

Native American Healing Methods

The primary idea behind Native American Healing is that when we face a difficulty, we should change our behaviors towards nature, other people, and, of course, ourselves. I've received Native American healing magic, and the fact is that it was terrifying. The practitioner told me that in order to be healed, I needed to be reborn, which meant that my old self had to die.

This is honestly scary ,Although he did not mean for me to kill myself, suicide and murder are both regarded grave sins in Native American Belief, as they are in most religions. The practitioner advised me to let go of some of my old behaviors. That's exactly what he meant.

Disclaimer: When we participate in healing ceremonies, spells, and rituals, we do it in conjunction with the guidance of our Medical Doctors. If our doctors tell us to rest and avoid doing anything, including casting a healing spell, we listen to them and do what they say. Modern medicine is capable of doing miracles. However, magic can assist us in this process.

Smudging is a popular Native American healing practice. Smudging is an ancient technique for cleansing and removing parasites from your aura that involves the use of smoke from sacred plants, herbs, and resins. Although smudging is most commonly associated with Sage smoke, other herbs or resins may also be utilized. For example, you can utilize frankincense smoke to lift your spirits.

Native American healing practices are varied and can differ greatly between tribes and communities.

Here are four sorts of healing rituals that are often used:

•**Sweat Lodge Ceremony:** Entering a tiny, enclosed structure (the sweat lodge) where heated rocks are put in a pit is part of this purifying process. Herbal-infused water is poured over the rocks, generating vapor and searing heat. Participants pray, sing, and go through a spiritual and bodily cleaning process. Sweat lodge ceremonies are thought to promote physical and mental healing.

•**Medicine Wheel Ceremony:** Medicine wheels are circular stone assemblages utilized in many healing ceremonies. Participants frequently congregate around the medicine wheel, which symbolizes the circle of life, the seasons, and the four cardinal directions. Prayer, meditation, and the use of herbs or other natural elements may be used in healing ceremonies held at these locations to restore balance and harmony.

•**Herbal Medicine and Plant-Based Healing:** Herbs and plants are frequently used for medical purposes in Native American healing. Healers, often known as medicine men and women, are knowledgeable about plant-based treatments and their healing abilities. To treat various ailments, these healers produce herbal concoctions, teas, or poultices, often mixing herbal therapy with spiritual rites and prayers.

•**Dance and Healing Rituals:** Certain tribes have unique dance rites, such as the Sun Dance or the Ghost Dance, that are said to have healing properties. These dances have intense physical and spiritual elements and might span many days. Fasting, dancing, and prayer may be used by participants to seek healing for oneself or their community.

•**Take a cleansing bath :** A simple ritual in which you use salts to purify your aura.
It is crucial to highlight that Native American healing practices are profoundly entrenched in spirituality and frequently incorporate a holistic approach, addressing physical, mental, and spiritual well-being. These rituals are sacred to their distinct tribes and are often carried out by members of the community who have specialized knowledge and roles. When learning or engaging in these rituals, it

is critical to respect their cultural significance and privacy.

2.2 HERB PROCUREMENT

High-quality herbs are high-quality herbs regardless of where they come from. It may be a local health food store, a tiny local farm, or even your neighbor's garden depending on where you live. Your community may even have a herb shop. You might be shocked to learn that your grocery store also carries high-quality herbs, particularly those sold as produce.

If you reside somewhere with restricted access to herbs, you should look for a trusted internet merchant.

You'll also notice that the cost of herbs varies dramatically depending on where you buy them. Cheaper isn't always better. Local small producers must frequently charge a greater price for their herbs and herbal products, but the quality is typically considerably higher.

Experiment with little quantities first to learn which producers have the highest quality; this will help you choose whether it's worth the money.

When sourcing herbs, keep the following factors in mind: soil quality, growing practices, and how the herbs are dried or processed.

If the soil where the herbs are cultivated is contaminated with heavy metals or other pollutants, the plant matter is likely to be contaminated as well. It's critical to know where the herbs were cultivated so you can tell if the soil was clean. This can be a problem for herbs grown anywhere, but especially in areas where soil pollution regulations do not exist.

Some larger herb retailers, such as Mountain Rose Herbs, test their herbs to make sure they are free of soil-based contamination.

You may be hesitant to buy herbs grown in urban farms, but don't dismiss them: Talk to the farmers and inquire about their soil. Most urban farms use clean soil and water filtration to ensure the safety of their produce.

Growing practices are also critical. How were insects dealt with? What type of fertilizer was applied? Were the herbs grown in a greenhouse or in the open air? Were they grown in soil or hydroponically? All of these things have advantages and disadvantages, but the end result is the same: If the herbs have a vibrant color and strong aromas and flavors, they are of high quality.

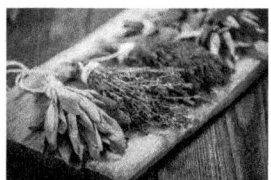 **Herbs**

The drying and processing steps can also be challenging: Herbs of high quality can be ruined if they are dried at too high a temperature or stored incorrectly. If there is significant browning in the dried herbs, you will know this is the case. This is the same browning that would be seen on a living plant with a brown, dried leaf—it appears un-vital.

Let's take St. John's wort as an example: This plant should have some brown when it's dried, but its brown color is a deep-red mahogany. That's considerably different from the brown-black color of basil leaves that have gone bad in your refrigerator. The latter is the one to avoid.

The basic thing is, know who you're buying your herbs from. Ask about their cultivation procedures, about the land and water, and about their processing practices. Not only does this help you make wise decisions, but it also helps build community between the people who farm our herbs (and food) and those of us who eat them. When we understand more about where our herbs originate from, we value them, our farmers, and our environment more.

2.3 HERB CULTIVATION

Planting a Native American herb garden is an excellent way to learn about and use native herbs. Native Americans collected plants that grew in locations where they settled or traveled through to eat and medicate themselves, dye cloth and materials, and smoke and burn for personal and spiritual purposes. Every region of the country had its own native herbs, but most of these herbs have now been cultivated in every region of the country, making them very easy to include into gardens everywhere.

You can grow your own herbs no matter how metropolitan your surroundings are. Many herbs will thrive in a pot under a sunny window - you don't even need a garden! If you've never grown a plant before, or if you've ever classified yourself as having a "brown thumb," don't worry: it's just like doing anything else. Spend a little time on it every day, and it will become second nature.

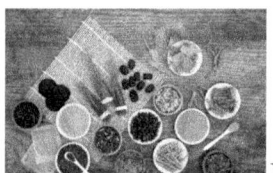 **Herbs**

Some herbs are unquestionably easier to cultivate than others. Mint, catnip, sage, and yarrow are simple to grow and may be purchased as seedlings or seeds from your local garden center. Mint and catnip are also very easy to grow indoors. If you don't have a garden or don't have safe soil to grow in, all are perfectly content to live in pots.

For roughly $15, you may have your soil tested by your local Extension Office, which will mail you a testing kit and provide results about soil safety as well as tips on the best type of fertilizer to use with the type of soil you have. The majority of the herbs you'll end up utilizing are worth growing yourself, and while true wildcrafting is the best option, it's time-consuming.

Here are some plants that you might want to try cultivating yourself. If you don't have a green thumb or the time to develop your plants from seeds or seedlings, they are usually relatively easy to grow from plants rather than seeds.

They are all pretty common and reasonably priced.
1. Garlic: antibiotic, stimulant
2. Rosemary: antioxidants that combat cancer, stimulant
3. Basil: antioxidants and anti-infection properties
4. Mint: a stimulant and digestive aid.
5. Lemon balm: a soothing tonic used to treat minor sadness, impatience, and anxiety.
Fennel has anti-inflammatory, analgesic, appetite stimulant, and anti-flatulent properties.

7.Lovage: anti-bronchitis, respiratory and digestive tonic

8.Oregano: antibacterial, antiflatulent, stimulates bile and stomach acid, and is antiasthmatic.

9.Cilantro (coriander): for flatulence, bloating, and cramps; as a breath freshener

10.Horseradish: stimulant, perspirant

11.Thyme: tea for altitude sickness prevention, antibacterial, inhalant (antiasthmatic), stimulant

The greatest method to get started with herbs, much like with herbalism, is to start! Purchase a seedling, place it in a pot with good soil and a little water, and keep an eye on it every day. Plants are living beings, and you'll learn to "hear" their communication in the same manner that you'll learn to interpret it.

Make A Native American Herb Garden

Native American herbs, like other herbs, demand well-drained, nutrient-poor soil that is not compact and slightly rocky. The herbs that aboriginal people collected might be found on sun-filled grasslands as well as deep in shade-filled forests, indicating that they could thrive in a variety of environments. Allow space for herbs to spread out and soil that has been well sifted and has a loose bed so that water may freely and rapidly drain. After you've made your bed, choose herbs based on what will grow best in your hardiness zone and the area you've provided.

2.4 HERBS PROCESSING

Medicinal plants are extracted and processed for direct ingestion as herbal or traditional medicine, or for use in research. Knowing how to appropriately prepare a herb in order to release the best therapeutic characteristics is part of the art of herbal medicine. Herbs have both internal and exterior use. When administered internally, they are usually more effective.

The four main internal preparations are decoctions, infusions, tinctures, and dry preparations.

The four basic external preparations are compresses, washes, salves, and poultices.

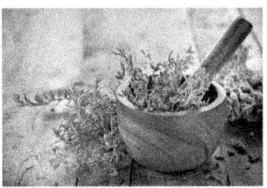

Herbal preparation and administration can be done and taken in a variety of ways; in traditional medicine, herbs were frequently prepared and provided as tea. These are referred to as decoctions or infusions. There are four major methods for efficiently preparing herbs, and they all work slightly differently depending on the potency of the plant and the desired result.

Water-based infusions and decoctions are the most popular preparations. Infusions are typically created from flowers and leaves, whereas decoctions are made from barks, roots, seeds, and berries.

An infusion is one of the most basic types of herbal preparation that many people are familiar with. Making a cup of tea is a fantastic illustration of infusion. The steps are similar: take a teapot, add dry herbs, a cup of boiling water, and let it set. It is best to consume infusions while they are hot. The decoction employs a lot more heat to remove the active ingredients from the plant's hard portions. You must place a teaspoon of plant materials in a saucepan. Powdered, shattered, or crushed into very little pieces. Then, bring a cup of water to a boil. When it reaches the boiling point, reduce the heat and leave it to simmer for around 15 minutes. While the mixture is still hot, drain and consume.

Infusions With Herbs:

The water method is used to make herbal infusions. Sugars, proteins, gums, mucilage, pectin, tannins, acids, coloring, mineral salts, glycosides, some kinds of alkaloids, and numerous essential oils are extracted using water. They should be utilized as soon as possible because they are not particularly shelf stable.

Infusions are typically made by revitalizing dried herbs, leaves, or flowers in hot water. We recommend using a non-metal teapot or saucepan to steep the materials you want to infuse in boiling water.

30g dried leaves/flower to 500ml boiling water is the recommended ratio.

Allow to steep for 20 minutes, covered. Drink while the ingredients are still hot/warm.

When using fresh herbs, the ratio should be 3 parts fresh to 1 part dried.

Decoctions - Decoctions involve a more difficult boiling procedure because the herbal materials typically consist of plant barks, roots, seeds, and stems. These, unlike leaves and flowers, are not easily infused. This process necessitates simmering/boiling down.

30g of ingredients to 750ml of water in a covered saucepan (no cast iron or aluminum) for 30 minutes to 1 hour or until half of the water has simmered down, for example, 750ml has simmered down to 500ml of liquid.

When using fresh herbs, the ratio should be 3 parts fresh to 1 part dried.

It is advisable to use ceramic or surgical grade stainless steel saucepans or teapots to ensure that nothing from the pot itself is incorporated into the finished product. It is preferable to avoid using cast-iron, aluminum, or synthetic-coated saucepans and teapots for this.

Herbal Tinctures:

A more complicated and slightly newer era way of herb utilization. Essential oils, resins, alkaloids, glycosides, organic acids, chlorophyll, acrid and bitter components, and castor oil can all benefit from a more stronger herbal extraction. This procedure is not indicated for removing minerals, gums, or mucilage.

A tincture is defined as the administration of an extract through the use of alcohol or another suitable vehicle.

Usual preparation entails soaking 60-120g of the herb in 500ml of 60-80 percent alcohol for 14 days, shaking once or twice every day. The herbs are separated from the alcohol after 14 days. To make a more potent tincture, press the mushy herbs through a cheesecloth to extract the leftover liquid. Once all of the liquid has been separated, it is placed in a dark amber glass dropper vial.

Because of the alcohol preservation, herbal tinctures can last for many years.

Please speak with your health care practitioner or Naturopath before utilizing any of these methods for the safest usage of the herbal characteristics as well as information on dosage and length of use specific to your needs.

•**Maceration:** This is an extraction method in which coarsely powdered drug material, such as leaves, stem bark, or root bark, is placed within a container and menstruum is poured on top until completely coating the drug material. After that, the container is sealed and maintained for at least three days.

The contents are swirled on a regular basis, and if placed within the bottle, it should be shaken occasionally to ensure complete extraction. The micelle is removed from the marc at the end of the extraction process using filtration or decantation. Following that, the micelle is separated from the menstruum through evaporation in an oven or on top of a water bath.This procedure is simple and ideal for thermolabile plant material.

•**Digestion:** This is an extraction method in which mild heat is used throughout the extraction process. The extraction solvent is put into a clean container, followed by the powdered drug substance. At a temperature of about 50o C, the mixture is placed over a water bath or in an oven. Throughout the extraction process, heat was used to reduce the viscosity of the extraction solvent and improve the removal of secondary metabolites. This approach works well with plant materials that are easily soluble.

•Percolation: The device used in this procedure is known as a percolator. It's a glass vase with a small cone form with holes on both ends. In a clean container, a dried, ground, and finely powdered plant material is soaked with the extraction solvent. A larger amount of solvent is added, and the mixture is maintained for 4 hours. The content is then put into a percolator with the lower end closed and allowed to stand for 24 hours.

The extraction solvent is then poured from the top down until the drug material is thoroughly saturated. The percolator's lower section is then opened, and the liquid is allowed to trickle slowly. A constant amount of solvent was introduced, and the extraction was carried out by gravity force, which pushed the solvent downward through the drug material.The solvent addition was halted when the volume of solvent added reached 75% of the total amount intended for the preparation. Filtration and decantation are used to separate the extract. The marc is then expressed, and the needed volume is obtained by adding the final amount of solvent.

•**Capsulation** - Because some herbs can taste downright terrible to the palate, drawing moisture and tasting bitter in the mouth, encapsulation of goods is usually the best option for this herbal use.

Herbs are often prepared by grinding the dried herb into a fine powder in a seed mill or mortar and pestle. These can then be placed in a veggie capsule or a gelatin capsule of your choosing. Keep these capsules in a cool, dry area, and if possible, store them in a dark place or in an amber-colored bottle.

Dosing guidelines for capsules: 3000mg or 3g of dried herb equivalent is commonly taken three times each day. (Remove this portion)

Typically, this much herb can be packed into each pill. Capsule sizes range from

#0 (400-450mg)

#00 (500-600 mg).

#000 = 650-850mg

HERBAL BIBLE BOOK 2

CHAPTER 1

1.1 HERBAL MEDICINE'S ESSENTIAL TOOLS

If you're new to the vast world of herbalism, selecting the correct instruments can be a difficult endeavor. This list was created to help keep things simple.

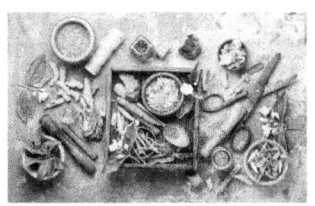

It is by no means comprehensive, but we hope it will get you started! With time, you'll be able to add to your arsenal of tools and herbs. When you combine that with expanding your knowledge through workshops and books, you'll be well on your way to being a true herbalist.

•Cheesecloth:

Cheesecloth, contrary to popular perception, is not only used to make cheese. Most seasoned herbalists' residences are likely to contain some cheesecloth. It acts as a strainer for various herbal preparations. It aids in the removal of every last drop of botanical goodness when producing herbal infused oils. The same holds true for straining tinctures, vinegars, and even nutritious herbal infusions. Look for unbleached organic cotton that is 100% organic. It's great to have around.

•Pestle and Mortar:

This collection of tools is useful for more than just looking like a herbalist, and you'll find that once you have one, you won't want to live without it! It comes in handy for producing spice blends with aromatic seeds like cumin or shattering fresh black peppercorns.

My daughter enjoys getting creative with the mortar and pestle and creating her own spice blends, sometimes with amazing success. I have even used it to break down roasted coffee beans in a pinch when my grinder finally gave out.

It's not only for dry spices, either. To make great pesto, use fresh herbs like basil, organic olive oil, and spices.

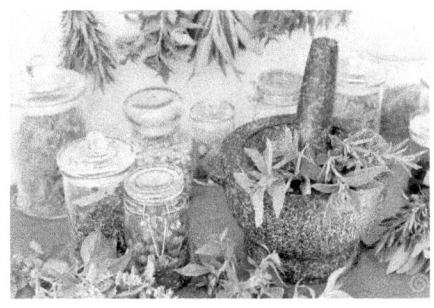

•Funnels:

Believe me, having a variety of funnels makes life better. I find funnels to be vital no matter how proficient one becomes at pouring liquid from one little bottle to another. They're well worth it because they save you from extra cleaning. You don't want to waste a single drop of the precious tincture you've been infusing and shaking on a daily basis.

I recommend purchasing a selection of sizes to accommodate a wide range of bottles. We also have one with a built-in strainer available. I also went to the brewery supply store and purchased a couple of extra large ones. I cannot recommend these highly enough for the new herbalist.

•Insertion of a Double Boiler:

A double boiler is essential for any recipe that calls for melting. While a glass jar or measuring cup can be used within a pot, I prefer to use a double boiler insert for convenience and safety. This useful addition nests in your sauce pan and features two pour spouts for easy transfer. I frequently use this instrument to melt wax and herbal oils in order to produce salves, creams, and lotions. This handy stainless steel component is easy to clean and can even go in the dishwasher.

•Screen for Sprouting:

I create alfalfa sprouts on a regular basis and add them to salads. In the spring, I like to collect dandelion greens and blend them with homegrown sprouts and a splash of homemade vinaigrette. Talk about frugal nutrition! However, this technique is useful for more than just sprouting. In fact, I believe sprouting screens are the most practical way to prepare healthy herbal infusions, which are one of my favorite ways to consume the benefits of herbs on a daily basis.

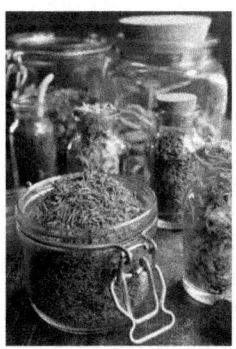

•Jars:

We adore our jars in all shapes and sizes, perhaps more than any other equipment in a herbalist's home. What else are we going to do with all of our organic herbs, spices, and teas? I have a jar for almost everything. I also use them to sip my own infusions instead of cups. You can never have too many jars .

•Dropper Bottles Made of Dark Glass:

Once you acquire a collection of these, you'll realize the importance of having funnels available. Dropper bottles made of amber or cobalt make it easy to enjoy your herbal compositions. They are specifically engineered to tolerate specific amounts of UV contamination, making them the appropriate storage solution for light-sensitive substances.

Fill these bottles with your herbal concoctions and give them as gifts to friends and family. Always remember to add a label at the end. It's a sad day when you have to flush that tincture down the toilet because you forgot to label the bottle.

1.2 USEFUL INSTRUMENTS FOR HERBAL MEDICINE

These tools make it easier to incorporate herbs into your life, especially if you have a hectic schedule, but they aren't as important as the ones listed above.

•**Grinder For Herbs:** For many years, a simple, little coffee grinder sufficed, but if you want to prepare a lot of herb powders, you may want to invest in a larger, dedicated machine.

•**Pressed Pot :** This is an insulated pot with a dispensing lever that you press.
People normally put coffee or strained tea in them, but we've found that placing herbs right into the pot, pouring in hot water, and letting it infuse works just as well. It will stay heated all day and can be dispensed by the cup. (Hold a small mesh strainer beneath the spout to catch any herb particles that fall down the tube.)

•**A Thermos:** A decent thermos is useful whether traveling or carrying tea to work. There are models with a filter integrated right into the lid, allowing you to put the herbs and water into the thermos together from the start.

•A French Press: This is our preferred method for creating herbal infusions. It allows the herb material to float freely in the water, exposes a large surface area for extraction (you simply press down to effortlessly dispense filtered tea), and is easy to clean.

1.3 NEEDED EQUIPMENTS

High-quality herbal medicines do not require expensive equipment or unique materials. The majority of stuff you'll need is most likely already in your kitchen.

•Jars Made Of Mason Jars: This is a herbalist's best friend. Because they're made of heat-resistant glass, you can prepare tea in them right away.
They're also useful for producing tinctures, keeping herbs, and other tasks. Quart and pint-size jars are the most adaptable, but larger jars may be necessary for storing dried herbs. Many store-bought goods

(such as sauerkraut and salsa) come in mason jars; simply hand wash or run through the dishwasher and dry to reuse.

•Strainers Made Of Wire Mesh: You'll need strainers of various sizes while straining tea or pressing tinctures. Begin with a couple single-mug strainers for preparing single cups of tea, as well as a bigger, bowl-size strainer for filtering greater amounts of herb-infused liquids.
Using cheesecloth. This is useful not only for straining and squeezing herbs in liquid, but also for wrapping herbs in a poultice.

•Cups And Spoons For Measuring : Cup, tablespoon, and teaspoon measurements are all useful, as are graduated measuring cups with pour spouts that may measure down to a quarter ounce.

•Conversion Funnels :A set of miniature funnels is highly useful for getting tinctures and other liquids into small-mouthed bottles.

•Bottles : Amber or blue glass bottles are ideal for keeping medicines over time. The "Boston round" shape is popular for tinctures and other liquid treatments, but any shape can suffice. Make a habit of saving and reusing any coloured glass bottles you come across—a number of kombucha brands, for example, come in amber glass.

Dose bottles are typically one or two fluid ounces in size, while storage bottles are often 4 to 12 fluid ounces. Use basic bottle caps for storage, but dropper tops are required for dosing bottles.
Labels . As soon as you manufacture your remedies, label them. Address labels are sufficient for most purposes; in a pinch, masking tape will do.

•**Using A Blender:** A normal kitchen blender will be enough for mixing lotions, breaking down bulky fresh plant stuff, and other tasks.

1.4 SAFETY RECOMMENDATIONS

Everything should be labeled. You can't be confident it's safe if you don't know what you're taking. Include information on all of the ingredients in the medicine as well as the date it was created.

•**Begin small** : When working with a novel medicine, start with tiny test batches and low doses. You may always increase your dose or take more later, but if a herb or preparation does not agree with you, it is advisable to start with a small amount.

•**Cautiousness:** Be cautious when using medications. Herbs and pharmaceutical pharmaceuticals (both prescription and over-the-counter) can interact in a variety of ways. This sometimes advantageous, positive herb-drug interactions may allow someone to reduce the amount of a drug or minimize its adverse effects but it is a complicated subject that should be handled with caution.

We identify the important interactions to look out for in the notes that accompany each remedy, but it's always better to speak with a practicing herbalist or your health care practitioner, especially if numerous medicines are being used at the same time.

•**Sensitivity:** Make use of your senses and always make sure to examine the herbs you're using as well as the end result. Examine your infused oil container for mold, and your dried herb package for remnants of packaging debris. Smell and taste your herbs and medicines to determine potency, and then dose accordingly.

•Make Only What You Require: If you find amazing benefits from a specific treatment and want to have it on hand every day, go for it. But no one needs a gallon of nasal spray solution, and it will go bad before you ever use it. Make exactly the medicines you require, and only as much as you require.

•Begin With What Is Plenty: You will most likely begin with herbs that are abundant in the wild or that are farmed commercially on a huge basis. As you expand your work with different plants, bear in mind those that are native to you and are not threatened or endangered. Don't be fooled into thinking that a rare, exotic herb is the sole one that can solve your problem.

CHAPTER 2

2.1 HERB PRESERVATION

Having a herb garden ensures that you always have the freshest, most delicious herbs on hand for culinary tasks. It also means having too many herbs to utilize all at once, which is a nice problem to have. We've all heard of drying herbs to save them for later use, but what about the herbs that are best utilized fresh? Can fresh herbs be preserved without being dried? Yes! Continue reading for an in-depth look at storing fresh herbs.

Key Takeaways:

Many home herb gardeners store their herbs without drying them in order to preserve the vibrant flavors that only fresh herbs can deliver.
Although freezing fresh herbs is the most common and efficient approach, there are numerous alternative ways to extend the flavor of fresh herbs.

What distinguishes fresh herbs from dried herbs?

Taste Herbs include naturally occurring chemical components that give them their distinct flavors. Some of these delicious molecules lose their power when herbs are dried, while others (cilantro, basil) just do not dry well. As a result, alternate preservation methods are the best approach to keep the flavor that these herbs lose throughout the drying process.

Nutrition and Aroma:

Herb aroma provides dimension to the meals and beverages we use them in, and dried herbs just do not have the same pungency as fresh herbs. The intense aroma left on your fingertips after pinching some fresh basil and the fragrance you get after opening a jar of dried basil are incomparable. The same chemicals that give plants their scent also contribute to their nutritional value. Other preservation procedures, such as freezing, tend to keep more nutrients than drying.

Dry herbs are wonderful in a variety of sauces and meals, but can you imagine muddling a dry herb for a cocktail or making pesto with dry leaves? Obviously not. There are many applications for herbs when a dried version just will not suffice.

How to Determine Which Method to Use

The honest truth regarding which method is best for preserving herbs is that, while certain herbs are best stored in particular ways, it all boils down to personal preference and how you intend to utilize the herbs afterwards. Dry herbs have hard, woody stems and tough leaves, but sensitive plants are better kept in other ways.

How to Keep Fresh Herbs

1. Temporary:

For short runs of a week or so, the easiest approach to extend the life of your herbs is to cut them at an angle with a sharp knife and store them immediately in a container of fresh water. This method is perfect for grocery store herbs that you want to keep fresh for more than a few days. It is feasible to keep herbs fresh for up to two weeks by changing the water every couple of days and refrigerating the bouquet.

2. Herb Freezing:

Freezing bare: The simplest way to freeze fresh herbs is to place them in a single layer on a baking sheet lined with parchment paper and freeze them. To begin, wash and dry the herbs before placing them on a baking sheet lined with parchment paper and freezing them. Once frozen, place them in a freezer bag or jar for later use.

Certain herbs with woody stems, like rosemary and thyme, freeze beautifully bare. Place the frozen sprigs in a bag and shake to separate the leaves from the stems. Then, remove the stems and store the leaves in a jar. Chives and lemongrass freeze beautifully this way as well: chop, freeze, and store. After being flash-frozen, the leaves will not stick together.

3. Create a Herbal "Cigar":

Many fragile, broad-leaved herbs do not do well when frozen bare. This variety of herbs freeze best when formed into a "cigar." Remove the leaves from the stems and place them in a freezer bag, pressing them into the bottom and then firmly rolling the bag, expressing all the air until you reach the top and close it. Place the plastic bag in the freezer, keeping it coiled up with elastic bands.

Remove the elastic bands, unzip the bag, and cut out only as much of the "cigar" as you need before refreezing the herbs. Cilantro, chervil, parsley, sage, tarragon, and other flat-leaved herbs work well with this method, which requires less freezer space than freezing loose leaves.

Ice Cube Freezing:

Certain highly fragile herbs that are best utilized fresh can be kept in the shape of ice cubes. Mint, cilantro, lemon balm, and other herbs can be kept in this manner for later use in recipes. Simply drop chopped or entire leaves into the cells of an ice cube tray, cover halfway with water, and freeze for about an hour.

Don't worry about the herbs floating to the top. Fill the tray to the brim with frozen vegetables and freeze again.Keeping the herbs totally enclosed in ice prevents oxidation and preserves their color and flavor. Transfer the frozen herb ice cubes from the tray to freezer bags or another sealed container for single-serving use as needed. Cubes can be put immediately into sauces or soups without needing to thaw. Herbed ice cubes can also be used to make cocktails, such as a mojito.

5. "Pesto" Cubes, Frozen:
Although basil is the most common ingredient in pesto, it is not the only one. When frozen bare, basil, oregano, marjoram, and many other herbs turn ugly and black. To keep these herbs at their most tasty and gorgeous, freeze them in an oil-based mixture.

Remove the leaves from the stems and pour a cup of fresh herbs into a blender or food processor with 1/4 cup olive oil and pulse until it is a good, homogenous mix. Pour the mixture into ice cube trays, then place in an airtight container for long-term storage. This method can also be used with whole leaves; simply press them into ice cube trays, cover with oil, and freeze.

6. Herbed Butter : Making herbed butter is a simple DIY technique to preserve fresh herbs for use in sautéing, spreading, or stuffing. Herbed butter is simple to create yet feels opulent.
To keep herbs in butter, use either salted or unsalted butter — the choice is entirely personal. Begin by

cleaning the herbs, then allow them to dry completely before separating the leaves from the stems. While the herbs are drying, soften the butter by leaving it at room temperature.

Finely mince the herbs and season with salt or lemon zest if desired. Mash the butter and herbs together in a mixing bowl until the mixture is perfectly homogeneous. Cut a square of parchment paper and spread all of the butter onto it using a spatula. Form a log out of the paper by rolling it around the mixture. Refrigerate it after folding the ends. Voila! You have herbed butter now.

This is a terrific way to add a little flair to your dish, and you can develop blends that are appropriate for different cuisines. Parsley butter with lemon zest brightens vegetables; basil butter enhances scrambled eggs or fish; sage butter accompanies chicken or biscuits; and herb combinations can perform a variety of culinary functions.

Almost any herb can be combined with butter. It will keep in the refrigerator for a few weeks but can also be frozen. Frozen herbed butter is best consumed within two months, although it can be stored for up to six months. Quality will degrade after that.

7. Herbed Salt:

For conscientious cooks, preserving herbs with salt is a truly rewarding method to preserve the season and add rich flavoring to savory dishes simply-with salt. The addition of garlic results in a perfectly balanced and dry-preserved spice blend that does not require a dehydrator or other specific equipment.

Begin with a half-cup of kosher salt, two cups of pungent fresh herbs--rosemary, thyme, savory, and sage are ideal--and four to five peeled garlic cloves. Mince the garlic with two teaspoons of salt in a food processor or with a chef's knife. Add the herbs to a food processor or chopping board and pulse until the mixture resembles coarse sand.

Spread the mixture on a baking sheet and top with the remaining salt. Allow it to cure in a sunny location near a window for a few days before transferring it to clean, dry mason jars. This salt is fantastic on popcorn, fried eggs, potatoes, and pretty much anything else. It's an excellent gift that can be saved for a year or more--if it lasts that long.

8 . Herbs Preserved in Salt:

Our forefathers knew how to preserve herbs without sophisticated apparatus, and salt-preserving was one of their favorite methods. This approach is ideal for delicate, sensitive herbs that dry poorly. Consider using this method to preserve basil, cilantro, chives, dill, parsley, or tarragon. You only need a clean, dry glass jar, fresh herbs, and kosher salt.

Begin by sprinkling salt in the bottom of the jar, followed by a single layer of herbs, then salt, and so on until the jar is full. Keep the jar in a cool, dark spot, such as a pantry shelf or even the refrigerator, and take out herbs as needed, shaking or rinsing off the salt if desired. When you're done with the herbs, the salt will still have the herb flavor and can be used in cooking or pickling. This method of preserving herbs should keep them fresh and usable for at least six months, but perhaps up to a year.

9. Herbed Sugar:

We far too often presume that herbs are only used for savory purposes in cooking. This is entirely unjust to plants, as proven by the following technique of storage: herb-flavored sugar. Layer fresh herbs with sugar to infuse the sugar with a delicate flavor and preserve herbs for separate use, using the same procedure as salt-preserving. It is also feasible to mince herbs into sugar using a food processor.

Consider mint, lemon balm, lavender, rosemary, thyme, or sage as herbs. Use the glass jar for baking, cooking, and drinks by storing it in a cold, dark spot or in the refrigerator. This method should keep herbs fresh for up to a year.

10 . Herbal Honey:

Honey is a natural preservative that is antibacterial, antifungal, and antiviral. It can also preserve the flavors of herbs for up to a year. To keep herbs in honey, choose local honey that is not overly flavored (some honey from seasonal flowers will have their own flavor).

Simply lay your herbs in a clean glass jar, whole or chopped, and top with honey. Allow the infusion to sit for at least six weeks to allow the flavors to fully penetrate before using to sweeten tea, as a syrup topping, in baking, or even as a basis for a meat glaze.

11. Infused Vinegar: Herb-infused vinegar isn't a new idea, but it's a simple method to keep the flavor

of your herbs for a long time and makes a great present. Begin with a lighter vinegar, such as champagne vinegar, white wine vinegar, or another light-colored vinegar.

Use clean glass canning jars and a small amount of herbs. Divide the sprigs evenly among the jars, then pour the vinegar over them, leaving at least a quarter-inch of space at the top. Screw on the lids and keep them in a cold, dark area for about a month. When you're ready to use the vinegar, strain it through a cheesecloth to eliminate any sediment.

Fill glass bottles halfway with vinegar and top with a decorative spring or two, if desired. These vinegars are excellent for salad dressings and marinades and may be stored indefinitely.

As you can see, there are numerous alternatives to drying to extend the life of your fresh herbs. Never again will a herb harvest or purchase go to waste.

2.2 MAKING SALVES

Herbal salves are a simple, effective, and practical method to consume herbal goodness! They are small enough to fit in a purse, pocket, or first-aid kit. Salves, while semi-solid at room temperature, soften when applied to the skin, making them less messy than oils.

They also make excellent gifts and are a simple and friendly method to expose newcomers to the healing power of herbs. Furthermore, salves can be made for a wide range of topical applications. Beeswax is added to protect, soothe, and nourish your skin.

Beeswax and oil are commonly used in salves. In reality, a simple lip salve can be made by blending warm olive oil and melted beeswax (approximately 5 parts oil to 1 part beeswax). As a first step in making a herbal salve (and incorporating the qualities and benefits of herbs), the oil is frequently infused with herbs.

Other substances, such as essential oils, vitamin E oil, lanolin, and glycerin, are frequently added to salves to improve their effectiveness. (Essential oils can offer smell, botanical, and aromatherapy benefits; vitamin E is regarded to be good for the skin and may help preserve the salve; lanolin makes the salve creamier; and glycerin adds moisture and may help prevent rancidity.)

Step 1: Produce Herb-Infused Oil

To begin making a salve, make your herb-infused oil(s). Depending on the method employed, this can take anything from a day to many weeks. If you're short on time or want to avoid infusing the oil yourself, you can buy infused herbal oils. We advocate using only dried herbs in your infusions because the lack of moisture in the plant material prevents spoiling.

Infusing your oil is the first step in preparing a herbal salve. There are various approaches to this.

No-cook Ways To Make An Herbal Oil Infusion

The heat of the sun can aid in the preparation of an infusion.
•Fill a glass jar halfway with herbs.
•Cover with oil, leaving about an inch of headspace.

•Stir, then leave the jar in the sun (outdoors or on a ledge inside if the weather is frigid) for three to four weeks. During this time, turn the jar over down every day or so.

•After the infusion period has expired, filter the oil via cheesecloth.

•Squeeze the cheesecloth to extract all of the oil, then discard (or compost, if possible) the herbs.

You can utilize your oil at this point, or (for a stronger infusion) repeat the procedure, putting the oil back in the jar with fresh herbs and leaving it in under the sun for about 4-5 weeks

Another no-cook approach is to keep the jar in a cold, dark spot (rather than in the sun) for six weeks. To spread the herbs through the oil, turn the jar over every now and then. When the timer goes off, filter the oil through the cheesecloth, squeezing the herbs as you go.

You can also infuse your oil in a slow cooker. Simply arrange your herbs in the bottom of the pot, cover with oil, and cook on low for eight hours. (Try this only if your pot has a low setting.) You may also put the herbs in a jar, cover with oil, and put the whole thing in the crockpot. (This method is useful for infusing multiple herbs in oils at the same time; simply place the jars in the crock pot next to each other.)

Method For Making An Herbal Oil Infusion On The Stove

Heat the dried herbs and oil (to cover) for about an hour over very low heat (a double boiler is useful to avoid burning). Turn off the heat and set the mixture aside for a few days. As a last step, strain through cheesecloth.

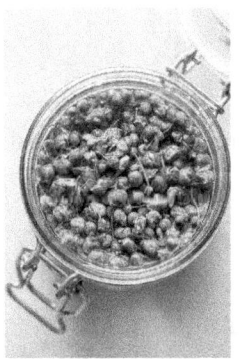

Step 2: How to Make Salve

After you've made your herbal oil, you're only a few steps away from having a finished salve.

In a saucepan, combine the infused herbal oil and beeswax (either beeswax beads or grated beeswax from a block) and slowly heat until the wax is melted. (Start with 1/4 cup of beeswax shavings or beads per cup of oil and modify as needed.) Remove from the fire and add the optional ingredients. Allow to cool in sterilized containers.

Some salve makers prefer to melt the beeswax in a separate pan before stirring it into the oil. Experiment to determine which technique you like.

The quickest way to make herbal salve combines the infusion and salve-mixing procedures. In a saucepan, combine your herbs and enough oil to cover. Simmer for around 30 minutes (do not overcook). Melted beeswax (approximately 1/4 cup per cup of oil) should be added to the oil. Allow to cool somewhat before straining through cheesecloth. If desired, add essential oils and other substances. Mix thoroughly, then pour into containers and put aside to set.

Pro tip: The consistency of salves can be readily altered to suit your tastes. Use less beeswax for a softer salve and more beeswax for a harder salve.Before making your salve, place a spoon in the freezer to test the consistency. When the beeswax has melted, spoon some salve onto one of the cold spoons and return it to the freezer for 1 to 2 minutes. This will be a simulation of the final consistency. Once the salve has cooled, you can modify the consistency by adding additional oil (for a softer salve) or more beeswax (for a harder salve).

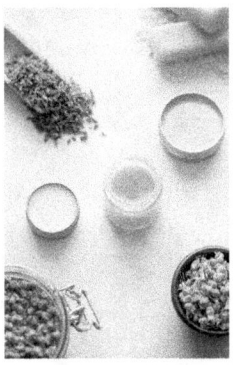

Salves' Best Herbs

Depending on your needs, you can produce a salve with a single herb or numerous herbs. It's a good idea to prepare a variety of herbal-infused oils so you can quickly make a salve when you need one.

Choose herbs that are appropriate for the goal of your salve. Saint John's wort,lavender, rosemary, marshmallow root, chamomile flower, calendula, goldenseal ,echinacea, mullein leaf and yarrow herb are among the most popular selections.

Before infusing the dried herbs in the oil, gently rub them between your palms. Allow fresh herbs to wilt for a couple of hours (on paper towels) to reduce moisture before using.
Olive, sesame, sunflower, coconut, sweet almond, and other skin care oils can all be utilized to produce your herbal infusion.
Combine more than one herbal infused oil in a single ointment for enhanced benefits.
Sterilize all of your containers and utensils before using them.

A double boiler is useful for preventing wax and herbs from burning, but a heatproof glass measuring cup inside a pan of water is also a choice.

Use only enamel or stainless steel pans, measuring cups, and spoons (no aluminum or Teflon). Stirring your recipe with wooden spoons is a fantastic idea.

Water encourages mold growth, so avoid getting even a drop in your salve (if using a double boiler, for example).

The consistency of your salve can be altered by adjusting the ingredient ratio.Using More beeswax makes a firmer Salve and more oil makes a softer salve.

To test the consistency, take 1 teaspoon of the oil/beeswax combination and blow on it or place it in the refrigerator until it solidifies. Try it out with your finger.

Before washing, wipe your pans and measure spoons with a paper towel. You don't want to get beeswax in your wash basin drain since it can solidify and plug it.

Even after washing, the beeswax will leave a film, so use old or designated salve-making pans and utensils.

Some essential oils, such as grapefruit and tea tree, may aid in the prevention of rancidity.

Salve will begin to harden as it cools (immediately), so pour it into your containers as soon as it's finished; don't leave it on the stove for too long.

Your salve should last around 6 months (or more if chilled).

Recipe For Herbal Salve

You don't need any special recipes to produce herbal salves. Simply select the herbs that best suit your needs and follow the instructions above. To get you started, here's a balm you might enjoy and find beneficial.

2.3 POULTICE

What exactly is a poultice?

Simply, a poultice is a convenient technique to apply herbal stuff to your skin. The herbs are combined with water, oil, or clay and applied in the form of a paste. The poultice is then wrapped in a cotton towel or gauze. To protect clothing, a waterproof cloth or layer of plastic wrap is often laid over the poultice, left on for several hours at a time, and changed a few times per day.

If the herb is extremely potent, such as garlic, ginger, or mustard, a small towel might be used to protect the skin before applying the herbal paste. The herbal cure could also be applied to the skin by placing it in a cotton bag. This can be accomplished by combining fresh or dried herbs with other helpful components.

A poultice is extremely advantageous because it keeps the damaged area of the body in constant contact with all of the plant's beneficial components for a lengthy period of time. Some herbs combat infection and inflammation, while others pull out poison and ease aches and pains. Poultices are commonly used to treat burns, boils, infections, inflammation, bruises, and aching muscles.

Some poultices can also be used to treat interior issues. Cold poultices can provide immediate relief from sunburn or insect bites. Making Your Own Poultice Perform a brief patch test before applying a poultice to rule out any skin allergies. Leave a small amount of the herb or oil you intend to use on the inside of your wrist or a non-irritated region of your skin for a few minutes.

Remove the material and wash the affected area with gentle soap and water if you observe any redness, itching, or other reaction. If nothing happens, you can apply the complete poultice to the affected region. Depending on your needs, there are numerous ways to make a homemade poultice.

A poultice is made by combining the entire herb or plant with oil, clay, charcoal, salt, or even simply water. Using your chosen ingredient, prepare the herb and make it into a thick paste. Traditionally, the fresh or dried herb is pounded into a paste with a mortar and pestle and blended with a liquid. I prefer to smash the herb using a granite mortar and pestle, although a blender or small food processor can also be used.

Depending on the potency of the herb, your thick paste can be applied straight to the problematic part of the body or wrapped between two layers of clean cloth before application. Cheesecloth or thin, organic cotton fabric are ideal for this since they allow the herbs to work their magic without allowing direct skin contact. However, it is also critical not to use a fabric that absorbs too much moisture.

Here's a quick guide to making your own poultice: Ingredients 2 to 3 teaspoons (or more as needed) of your favorite fresh or dried herbs, medicinal clays, oils, or activated charcoal. Sufficient amount of hot water to make a thick paste Covering with organic cheesecloth or cotton cloth A waterproof cover to keep the poultice in place. Crush the plant and combine it with the clay, oil, charcoal, salt, and water to produce a thick paste.

If you use an oil, you won't require as much water, if any at all. Flour can also be used to thicken the paste. Apply the paste to the skin directly or distribute it between two layers of cloth and apply it to the affected area. Secure with more cloth, gauze, plastic, or waterproof fabric. If you want to warm up the poultice, place it on a heating pad. As needed, leave the poultice on for 30 minutes to 3 hours and repeat.

Recipes for Four Favorite Poultices These are our top four poultice recipes for a variety of diseases and conditions.

1. Mustard seed poultice for a sore throat or cough Begin by crushing the mustard seeds or using a high-quality mustard seed powder. Combine your mustard, flour, and warm water to make a thick paste. Because mustard seed is quite strong, it is best to apply it to the chest or back by spreading the paste between two layers of fabric.

2. Poultice of frankincense and myrrh for bruises and skin swelling Allow 24 hours from the time of damage before applying the poultice to the bruised or swollen region. To thicken the mixture, combine the organic essential oils of frankincense and myrrh with either organic olive or sesame oil and some flour or honey. Cover the area with plastic wrap after applying the paste. For around 30 minutes, place a heating pad on top of the poultice.

3. Castor oil poultice for menstrual cramps To begin, combine organic castor oil with moxa essential oil (derived from the mugwort herb). Add flour or honey to the mixture to make a paste. Place an

organic cotton rag on the lower belly and apply the paste. Put your feet up, eat some dark chocolate, and unwind for about 25 minutes.

4. Arthritic pains, joint discomfort, and carpal tunnel syndrome: ginger or turmeric poultice When used as a poultice, ginger and turmeric are potent antioxidant herbs that can efficiently permeate the skin. These two herbal medicines can be utilized to treat deeper layers of inflammation in hurting body areas.

Make a paste with ginger powder or turmeric powder and a small amount of warm water. Cover the affected region with a cheesecloth and apply the paste. For around 20 minutes, place a heating pad on top of the poultice. If you choose turmeric, be in mind that it may briefly tint your skin yellow. Turmeric and ginger each have blogs, so be sure to check them out.

In conclusion Poultices are one of our favorite (and safest) ways to get the benefits of herbs' mystical abilities. They can be administered straight to the skin and are used to treat a range of ailments. Poultices have all of the advantages of herbs but are less concentrated than tinctures or oils. Because herbal poultices are topical medicines, you should avoid using them on or near an open wound or eczema to avoid any unfavorable reactions.

2.4 SMUDGING

Smudging is a Native American ceremony that connects smoke and spirituality in extraordinary ways.

This is a popular ceremonial rite practiced by indigenous peoples to purify, spiritually cleanse, clear physical regions of negative energy, and bless. Continue reading if you are a Native American or simply want to learn more about Native American culture to broaden your views.

Smudging is a practice practiced by many Indigenous societies that entails the burning of one or more of these remedies. Smudging can be done in a variety of ways, with many variants and methods.

Smudging enables people to come to a halt, slow down, and become more conscious and centered. This enables people to recall, connect with, and remain grounded in the event, task, or purpose at hand.

Smudging also aids in the release of unpleasant emotions and thoughts. The feeling of being quiet and protected during smudging encourages people to let go of things that keep them from being balanced and focused.

Smudging is always optional. It is perfectly appropriate to signal that you do not want to smudge. That person can either stay in the room and not smudge or leave the room during the smudge. Any Indigenous tradition's guiding value is respect for all.

What Exactly Is Native American Smudging?

To truly grasp the concept and undertake this ancient rite yourself, it's vital to first understand what exactly smudging comprises. Smudging is defined as a ceremony that involves burning plant herbs and resins in a clay or shell bowl while praying. This causes a smoke cloud to form, which is thought to cleanse the air and people who breathe it.

Smudging is, in fact, the most common technique performed to cleanse people and places of negative energy that they would rather not be exposed to. Smudging is practiced by numerous Native peoples in the Western Hemisphere and has been for generations.

Why Do Smudging Rituals Take Place?

There are various reasons why someone may choose to smudge, but the most common is to improve the lives of people and the environments in which they live. Smudging serves as a conduit between mortal existence and the higher realms, bringing in good spirits while expelling any negative, stagnant ones. After the cleansing, this ceremony removes any grief, impurities, and fears, as well as improves health, leaving nothing but serenity and harmony for both humans and the environment.

Which Herbs Should I Use?

Before we get into the act of smudging and how it's done correctly, let's go over the herbs used for smudging so you're fully prepared to either try it yourself or get the broader picture. For example, most herbs used to smudge contain antibacterial properties, which means that when burned, they truly clear the air.

Two white sage smudge sticks, two palo santo sticks, an abalone shell bowl, and a rose quartz crystal are included in this smudging package.

Sage is a healing herb that includes both Salvia Apiana (white sage) and Salvia Officinalis (common sage). "Salvia" is derived from the Latin word "salvare," which means "to feel healthy, well, and healing." Both white and common sage are used to provide strength, clarity, and wisdom, and they both reflect the maternal lineage of women.

Cedar - Cedar is renowned for cleaning and purifying, removing evil spirits from people and items in order to restore harmony. Burning cedar is also used to generate happiness and to deepen human connections to the spiritual worlds

Sweetgrass - Known as Mother Earth's hair, sweetgrass is widely used by all Native Americans and is said to transport prayers into the spirit world. It is stated that the smoke from the herbs takes the words and transitions them. It is also known as "holy grass" because when it burns, it produces a pleasantly fragrant haze rather than an open flame.

Tobacco is a very sacred medication in many cultures and is widely regarded as the ideal link between the human and spiritual realms. It does not have to be smoked in order to bring spiritual advantages. This is used to demonstrate thankfulness for the beauty in life as a human commitment established and supported by the spiritual realm.

Though these are the most popular herbs used to begin, conduct, or end a smudging ritual, essential oils are also used. Wormwood,Mugwort Lavender,Yellow Birch,Carrot seed,Thuja Oil,Balsam Fir oil, Juniper Berry, and Peppermint are among them. Now that we've covered the essentials, it's time to grab your herbs and other smudging supplies and get started. Gather the following items to begin your group circle or private session:

An abalone shell, clamshell, or huge clay bowl

Choose your own herbs, but remember to remove the stems.

Matches made of wood

To wave the smoke, use large feathers or smudge sticks (or your hands).

Once you've completed all of this, it's time to get started. If this is your first time doing this, I recommend performing a session on your own to fully get the hang of it and the feeling it provides. There are various methods to do this sacred ceremony on your own, but here is a simple one you may do at home to practice with.

If you are performing this ceremony indoors, make sure to open a window to ensure adequate airflow. Remember, the aim is to get some smoke, but you don't want to become sick from it or set off your smoke alarms.

Make certain that you are fully present and focused. If you are distracted in any manner, the smudging procedure will be unsuccessful or will not operate as well as it might.

Light the match and ignite the herbs in the bowl for 20 to 30 seconds before extinguishing the fire by placing your hand above it to deprive it of oxygen (using your breath to blow it out is not correct).

The herbs in the bowl will begin to emit smoke. Smudge yourself first with the feather or smudge sticks (head first to your feet), then move to your surroundings. Make care to cover every corner and item gently and relaxedly.

When you're finished, take the ashes from the herbs outside and replace them in the soil. This represents the return of energy to the earth and expresses respect.

Burning Sage For Smudge

As you can see, burning plants like sage and cedar has far more significance than simply creating a cloud of smoke while uttering a prayer.

Native Americans historically believed that the power of herbs and healing were the best ways to rid the body or environment of undesired ideas, feelings, spirits, and negative energy in order to achieve a greater state of well-being. Indigenous cultures have a strong connection to Mother Earth and utilize the gifts she has provided to heal and create beneficial effects. Despite the fact that times have changed and the world has grown more modernized than ever, smudging is still a widely practiced ceremony that is vital to Native American culture today, deserving of the highest attention and respect.

HERBAL BIBLE BOOK 3

CHAPTER 1 : THE WHEEL

1.1 GLOSSARY OF NATIVE AMERICAN TRADITIONS

•The Ghost Dance

The Ghost Dance was a religious movement among the Plains and Rocky Mountain Indians. It began in 1870, when a Paiute prophet named Wodziwob had a spiritual vision in which he saw the dead revived, wild wildlife returned in their former quantities, and traditional Native lifeways restored. The Paiutes' neighbors in the Great Basin and Northern California participated in the vision-required circle dance in order to bring these things about. Following the vision of another Paiute prophet named Wovoka in 1890, the Ghost Dance was revived and extended even more, expressing both the hope and desperation of the Native peoples.

•Ceremonies for Green Corn

Green corn rites have long been a part of the ritual lives of Native American tribes in the southeastern United States. These agricultural rites honor the New Year and the regeneration of all life by celebrating the ripening of the maize harvest. Homes and public spaces are thoroughly cleaned, all fires are extinguished, and old food is consumed. To honor the regeneration of all life, the New Year begins with a priest gently igniting a new flame and offering the first of the growing maize. A feast and dance follow.

•Leader in Medicine

A shamanistic spiritual leader in one of the Native American traditions is referred to as a "medicine man" in English. Although most experts believe the phrase to be obsolete because it only relates to one part of the activity of these ritual officiants, it is nevertheless widely used by the general people.

•Myth

Myths are stories that humans tell about the nature of reality: how the order of things we know came to be and how it operates on the basis of deep truths. Myths can be about creation events, divine dramas involving God or the gods, or the discoveries and struggles of superhuman ancestors. In any event, myths do not serve to impart historical or scientific fact since the truth they hold is a deeper truth that orients humans in the universe and bases their fundamental values.

•Native American

Each of the many Native American nations has its own particular way of life, yet some qualities are shared by all. The majority of Native life-ways are predominantly taught orally; they are geared towards living in relation to a specific terrain; and they share a vital interest in the spirit world, visionary and dream experience, and the transformational power of music and dance.

•Church of the Native Americans

Native American spiritual and ritual practices involving the sacramental ingestion of hallucinogenic peyote are combined with Christian teachings in the Native American Church. Visions are sought not for their own sake, but for the significance they may offer for healing and guidance in everyday life. Its four-part ethical code comprises brotherly love, family duty, self-reliance, and alcohol abstinence. The Native American Church is the country's largest Native religious organization.

•Peyote : is the common name for the cactus Lophophora williamsii, which the Aztecs called peyotl. The hallucinogenic cactus buttons are ritually gathered and consumed by diverse Native Americans. The Native American Church combines peyote ingesting ceremonies with Christian traditions.

•Pipe Ceremony
Many Native American peoples rely on the sacred pipe for spiritual and cultural survival. Each component of the pipe—stem and bowl, tobacco, breath, and smoke—represents fundamental interactions that keep the universe in motion. During ceremonies, many pinches of tobacco are used to symbolize requests for blessings on behalf of all of creation. The prayers become visible offerings when

they are lit by the fire of the Great Spirit and inhaled and expelled as smoke.

powwow

•**A powwow :** is a Native American gathering of dancing, singing, drumming, and socializing that is more about celebration than ceremony. They are now a key manifestation of an intertribal Native American identity that supplements tribal identities. Every year, over 900 powwows are hosted across the United States and Canada.

•**The Sun Dance:**

The Sun Dance is a purification and regeneration ceremony frequently practiced by Native American Plains tribes. Although the many Sun Dance rites differ in many respects, they all entail a grueling marathon of dancing oriented around a center pole in a lodge specially constructed for the sun dance .Self-mortification and fasting are also common in dance rites, and are frequently accompanied by strong visionary experiences. Such rites are thought to help refill the creation, refresh the spiritual vigor of those who participate, and benefit humanity as a whole.

•Sweat Puddle:

The Native American sweat lodge is a lashed construction of bent poles covered with blankets, skins, or tarps to keep the heat in, which is given by hot stones brought into the lodge. Those who enter the lodge offer their prayers while pouring water over the stones. The steamy sweat lodge rites are performed for purification, healing, and well-being. The sweat lodge, in one form or another, is an important component of the lives of many Native Americans across North America, from Alaska to the Great Plains to the Eastern Woodlands.

•Quest For Vision:

Vision quests are a typical way for Native Americans to establish touch with the spirit world and seek the guidance of a specific manifestation of divine power. The quest is sometimes associated with becoming adulthood, but it can occur at any time when spiritual discernment is required. Following preliminary purification procedures, one would travel to a remote location, particularly one of the many sacred sites linked with vision quests, such as the Black Hills of South Dakota or the Medicine Wheel in Montana's Bighorn Mountains. The three or four day experience includes fasting and prayer while remaining alert to signs and dreams that disclose a vision.

1.2 THE NATIVE AMERICAN MEDICINE WHEEL

Native Americans have a strong connection to nature, which is used to develop and preserve balance, health, and wellness. Nature is referred to as "Mother Earth," and her significance has been incorporated into a variety of customs and traditions. The medicine wheel, which depicts both perfection and the circle of life, is one example of this philosophy.

Most medicine wheels, also known as holy hoops, contain four common compass points, each with its own guiding spirit, that represent the four stages of life and offer lessons and gifts to aid in the formation of a balanced life.

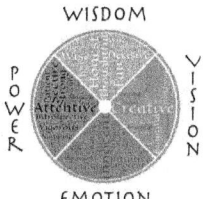

Medicine Wheel

The four points may also have animal, botanical, celestial, and other representations that vary considerably amongst tribes. For example, the buffalo that occurs on Plains Indian medicine wheels is not portrayed on the wheels of southern tribes because that animal was uncommon among them, and an alligator would not show on the medicine wheels of northern tribes.

Many Native American tribes revere the number four because it signifies the four seasons, the four human needs (physical, mental, emotional, and spiritual), the four kingdoms (animal, mineral, human and plant, and so also the sacred medicines (four) (sage,sweet grass,tobacco and cedar)

The Medicine Wheel can take several shapes in many types of artworks or as a physical structure on the ground. Medicine Wheels have been created on Native American sites for thousands of years.

The Bighorn Medicine Wheel, located in Wyoming's Bighorn National Forest, is one of the most noteworthy. For years, Crow adolescents have utilized this sacred location for fasting and vision quests, while other Native Americans have used it to give gratitude and pray.

The Medicine Wheel was named by white explorers who discovered it near the end of the nineteenth century. This wheel, the most southern and largest in existence, is claimed to function as a form of signpost to locate the sunrise of the summer solstice. In its most basic form, the Medicine Wheel represents all of creation, including all races of humans, birds, fish, animals, trees, and stones. It has the shape of a waggon wheel and is built of stones.

The circular shape of the wheel, according to tribal beliefs, depicts the earth, the sun, the moon, the cycles of life, the seasons, and the transition from day to night. The rotation path of the earth is followed by moving around the perimeter of the Medicine Wheel in a clockwise fashion. Creator sits perfectly balanced in the center of the wheel, at the hub. An inner circle outside the center represents the Old Woman (the earth), Father Sun, Grandmother Moon, and the four elements.

On the perimeter, four unique rock mounds were set in the four directions, divided by stones depicting the moon's cycles. Stones arranged in straight lines from the periphery to the center (the spokes of the wheel) signify spiritual routes that bring us to the center, to perfect balance, to the Creator.

Other stone Medicine Wheels can be found over the plains of Alberta and British Columbia, Canada, as well as the northern United States.

Four Directions Prayer...

Great Spirit of Light, come to me with the force of the rising sun from the East (red). may there be light in my words, and may there be light on my road. Let me always remember that you give the gift of a new day. And never let me be plagued with regret for not starting afresh.

Come to me, Great Spirit of Love, with the force of the North (white). Make me brave when the chilly wind blows on me. Give me courage and endurance for everything that is harsh, painful, or causes me to squint. Allow me to go through life prepared to accept whatever comes from the north.

I face West (black), the direction of dusk, Great Life-Giving Spirit. Allow me to remember every day that the time will come when my sun will set. Never let me forget that I have to blend with you. Give me a lovely color, a great sky for setting, so that when the time comes for me to meet you, I can come in glory.

Send me warm and relaxing winds from the south (yellow), Great Spirit of Creation. When I'm tired and cold, please comfort and caress me. Unfold me like the soft breezes that blow through the trees' leaves. Give to me your warm, moving breeze, like you do to the rest of the land, so that I may grow close to you in warmth. Man did not weave the tapestry of existence; he is merely a strand within it. Man does to the web what he does to himself.

How To Make A Medicine Wheel

For millennia, ceremonial circles have been utilized to improve spiritual experiences. The medicine wheel is a traditional spiritual practice among Native Americans, with each direction of the wheel signifying an energy or force in nature or the spiritual realm. Medicine wheels are often made with stones, but they can also be made with jewelry, ribbons, feathers, sea shells, and bundled plants. The objects reflect characteristics of yourself as well as the factors that guide your life.

1. Decide where you want to put your medicine wheel.

Choose a spot for your medicine wheel. Choose a location where you will feel comfortable and able to meditate once the wheel is complete. This position could be inside or outside.

2. Collect the objects

Collect the items you want to use for your wheel. Each direction requires four objects: north, south, east, and west. Place a fifth object in the centre of your circle. This is your connection to the spirit realm, the soil, and your ancestors.

3. Locate the center

Find the center of the circle you want to make. Insert a stick into the ground and push down to secure it. Find true north with a compass and place one object in the path straight north of the stick. Place another object to the east, equidistant from the center as the object to the north. Repeat the process for the west and south directions.

4. Take out the stick

Take out the stick and center the fifth object. To bless the medicine wheel, perform the ceremony of your choice. Using the medicine wheel, meditate according to your belief system.

5. Colorize your medication wheel.

Colorize your medicine wheel as desired. Colors can be utilized for items positioned in either direction. The center object can be an object with all of the colors or a single color representing the notion on which you want to meditate.

6. For the east, use a red object.

For the east, use a red object. This color is associated with the sunrise and new beginnings. Red objects should be placed in the south to represent fire and desire.

7. Make use of a yellow object.

Use a yellow object to indicate healing and growth in the south. Place it in the east for new beginnings and change.

8. Put a dark item there.

To depict reflection and meditation, place a black object to the west. Black in the west signifies an investigation of the past and preparation for your life's winter.

9. stands for ancestral wisdom and spiritual direction.

A white object placed to the north represents ancestral wisdom and spiritual direction. A green item in the north can also symbolize your commitment to the Earth as your mother.

The cardinal directions of north, south, east, and west correspond to elements, colors, and healing characteristics. While conventional depictions of the directions exist, each individual should consider what the direction means to them in respect to their location in the world. For example, if a pagan practitioner lives in an area where water is to the east, east may represent water to them.

1. North

The element earth is related with the direction north in pagan religions. Rocks, clay, soil, salt, and sand are examples of it. One of them is commonly used to mark the direction north in a pagan circle. Other associations with north include the color green, physical power, and the pagan symbol of the pentagram. A pagan may place a dish of salt to the north when casting a circle.

2. South

In Pagan beliefs, the direction south is related to the element of Fire. In Pagan rites, physical fire, as well as lightning, electricity, and candles, symbolize the southern direction. The color red and the pagan wand or staff are also associated with the south.The south direction is invoked for the sake and reasons of inner fire and passion. A pagan may place a lit candle to the south when casting a circle.

3. East

In pagan traditions, the element air is usually connected with the direction east. During pagan rituals and rites, the East is represented by feathers, chimes, or incense. The color yellow and the pagan athame or dagger are both associated with the east. The East is summoned for issues of intellect and the human mind. A pagan may light incense in the eastern quarter when casting a circle.

4. West

Water is the element most commonly linked with the direction west. Shells and water are emblems of the west in Pagan beliefs. The color blue and the tool of a chalice or cup are frequently used in Pagan traditions to signify the west. The West is called for intuition and feeling. When casting a circle, the western quarter is frequently ornamented with a water chalice.

5. Center

The element of spirit is represented by the center in Pagan beliefs. White is connected with the center. Goddess depictions present the center of ceremonies and rituals. The color white is another way to depict the center. The center is evoked for reasons of spiritual connection, dream work, and inner self. When casting a circle, a goddess symbol might be placed in the center.

●

1.3 THE SACRED PIPE CEREMONY

For First Nations people, the pipe is extremely sacred. It was once used to start discussions between different nations in order for positive talk to take place. This ritual was also seen as a method for participants to be truthful, respectful, and to follow through on the decisions and commitments made during the meeting period. Tobacco that has been blessed by prayer is typically used in the ceremony.

The pipe is typically stored in a sacred bundle owned by the pipe carrier, and only he (or a helper) is permitted to open the bundle in preparation for the ceremony. The ceremony can begin once all preparations have been completed. When asked, the pipe carrier can perform the ritual practically anywhere.

The participants form a circle around the pipe carrier. In some First Nations, men sit in an inner circle and women in an outside circle; in others, everyone sits in one circle. Women who are in their menstrual period are not permitted to participate in this ritual since it is considered that they have immense power and could harm the ceremony. The assistant inserts the sacred tobacco into the pipe and fires it in front of the pipe carrier.

The ceremony's host, the pipe bearer, prays to seven cardinal points: the Four Directions, the Above or Spirit World, the Below or Mother Earth, and the Centre or all living things. The pipe is then handed around to the participants, who can either touch it or smoke it. The pipe's passage can be repeated multiple times. After allowing the tobacco to "die," the pipe is disassembled and returned to the bundle until the next ritual.

Following this, the pipe carrier may say a few words of thankfulness regarding life and expectations; each participant is then invited to say a few words of gratitude; and the ceremony is regarded as closed.

The pipe is immensely sacred to First Nations people. It was originally utilized to start dialogues across different cultures in order for constructive conversation to occur. This ritual was also viewed as a way for participants to be truthful and courteous, as well as to follow through on decisions and pledges made during the meeting session. In most cases, prayer-blessed tobacco is used in the ceremony.

The pipe is usually kept in a sacred bundle possessed by the pipe carrier, and only he (or a helper) is allowed to access it before the ceremony.

Once all preparations have been done, the ceremony can begin. When summoned, the pipe bearer can perform the ritual almost anywhere.

A circle is formed by the participants around the pipe carrier. Men sit in an inner circle and women in an outer circle among some First Nations; in others, everyone sits in one circle. Women in their menstrual period are not permitted to participate in this rite because they are thought to have enormous power and could disrupt the event. The pipe carrier's assistant inserts the sacred tobacco into the pipe and ignites it in front of him.

The pipe bearer, the ceremony's host, prays to seven cardinal points: the Four Directions, Above or Spirit World, Below or Mother Earth, and Centre or all living things. The pipe is then passed around to the participants, who have the option of touching it or smoking it. The passage of the pipe might be repeated several times. After allowing the tobacco to "die," the pipe is disassembled and placed back in the bundle until the next ritual.

Following that, the pipe carrier may offer a few words of thanks for life and expectations; each participant is then invited to say a few words of thanks; and the ceremony is considered closed.

1.4 SWEAT LODGE

Indigenous peoples in Saskatchewan and throughout North America. It is a purifying ceremony that can be done alone or as a precursor to other ceremonies like the Sun Dance. The location of the resort is usually chosen with care. A fire pit is dug, and specifically selected rocks are heated. These rocks range in size from 25 cm to 50 cm and can retain heat for an extended period of time.

A trench is then dug in the heart of the site where the lodge will be built to retain the hot rocks during the ceremony. The builder then gathers supple saplings that are bent to make a dome; for many First Nations, this dome signifies Mother Earth's womb. Layers of blankets are used to cover the saplings, and canvas tarpaulins are occasionally used to cover the blankets (furs and bark were previously used). The lodge's entrance is normally facing east.

When the ritual is set to begin, one person will remain outside to supervise the hot rocks and place them in the central pit during the ceremony.

The ceremony is normally held in the late afternoon and can linger until daybreak the next day. There are two styles: one with merely heated rocks and one with water poured on the rocks. Both will provide the desired sweat effect. When the rocks are sufficiently hot, the participants strip naked or wear only light undergarments. The host then enters the lodge on his hands and knees, followed by the others, who sit in a circle around the center pit. When all of the participants have entered the lodge, the fire-tender begins to pass the heated rocks into the pit.

The number of rocks used ranges between sixteen to sixty-four. The number and placement of the rocks are just as significant as the whole ceremony; each First Nation will emphasize different components based on their needs. The entry is closed and the host begins to pray after a number of heated rocks are passed into the Lodge.

During this moment, participants are free to pray in their own style. To avoid any health risks, everyone leaves the lodge for a while and then returns. Depending on the needs of the participants, this process might be repeated up to four times. Everyone wishes everyone else a happy life at the end of the ceremony. Following the ceremony, the host's family will generally hold a customary feast.

Getting Ready To Build Your Own Sweat Lodge

There are a few important measures to take before making your own Sweat Lodge. To begin, it is critical to select the appropriate site. An isolated spot in nature away from the hustle and bustle of daily life is excellent. Second, obtaining the required supplies is critical. Natural materials such as willow branches, blankets, and tarps are examples of this. Preparing for the ceremony is equally important.

A Sweat Lodge ceremony is a spiritual experience that must be approached with reverence and mindfulness. Understanding the significance of the ritual can be aided by learning about the history and advantages of Sweat Lodges. Check out the link to

Shaman Sweat Lodge Analysis for a more in-depth analysis of Sweat Lodge ceremonies.

•Selecting a Location

The location of your sweat lodge is critical for creating a safe and comfortable experience. When choosing a place, keep in mind that sweat lodges must be built on flat ground, free of waste and plants. To minimize flooding, the region should also have sufficient drainage. Other factors to consider when selecting a place for your sweat lodge include:

Factors to Consider

•**Accessibility:** Select a good accessible location, riverine area is of great importance This will make constructing and operating your sweat lodge easier.

•**Privacy** : Choose a quiet location where you will not be disturbed. This will contribute to a feeling of solitude and intimacy during the ceremony.

•**Nature proximity** : Look for a site that is close to nature and has little noise from traffic and other human activity. This will contribute to a sense of calm and connection to the natural world.

•**Sunlight Exposure :** Consider where the sun will be during the day and select a place that will provide ample shade during the warmest parts of the day.

•**Windy conditions :** Consider the direction and strength of the prevailing winds and select a site that provides some wind protection.

An isolated and scenic area with level ground, excellent drainage, and easy access to water will be ideal for your sweat lodge. You're laying the groundwork for a safe and transformative experience by choosing the perfect location for your sweat lodge.

•**Getting Supplies:**

There are a few crucial items you'll need while gathering ingredients for your own sweat lodge. To begin, you will need a huge piece of canvas or tarp to cover the lodge. This will assist in keeping the heat and steam inside. You'll also need long, straight branches or saplings to build the lodge's frame.

These branches should be strong enough to hold the weight of the canvas/tarp while still being thin enough to bend and mold into a dome-like structure. If you're not sure where to look, a local hardware store or landscaping business might be able to assist.

You'll also need a few smaller supplies in addition to these primary materials. Rocks are an important part of a sweat lodge ceremony because they are heated and used to generate steam inside the lodge. For this, you'll need many huge, heat-resistant boulders. These are normally available in a landscaping or construction supply store.

You'll also need blankets, towels, and pillows for seating and comfort during the ceremony. It's also a good idea to keep a bowl of water available for participants to sip or use as a cooling device. For a more sensual experience, some individuals add herbs or other fragrances to the water.

Finally, gather any additional objects that you might require for the specific type of sweat lodge ceremony you'll be hosting. If you're following a Native American tradition, for example, you might require special sacred herbs or prayer objects to use during the ceremony. Make sure to complete your study ahead of time and obtain all of the necessary supplies.

Checklist of Supplies:

•Canvas/tarp

•Saplings/branches

•Heat-resistant large rocks

•Throws, towels, and pillows

•A water bowl

•If relevant, sacred herbs or prayer objects

Remember to take your time acquiring supplies and double-checking that everything is in order before starting construction. You'll be well on your way to creating your own customized sweat lodge with the correct resources and a clear plan of action.

If you want to learn more about the distinctions between sweat lodges and saunas, read this article. You can also learn more about the science underlying sweat lodge ceremonies in this related topic. While sweat lodge ceremonies can be powerful and transformational, it's also vital to recognise the controversy that surrounds these practises. More information about these topics can be found in our article here.

Constructing Your Sweat Lodge:

Building your own sweat lodge can be difficult, but with the correct materials and careful preparation, anyone can build a holy area for a sweat ritual. Construction must be done step by step to ensure the safety and functionality of your sweat lodge. To begin, dig a shallow pit in the center of your chosen area in which you will ignite a fire to heat the stones.

To produce the dome shape, build a structure from flexible branches like willow or hazel and cover it with blankets, hides, or tarps. Tightly close the covering to prevent air from entering and interrupting the ceremony.

Finally, create a flap or aperture on the side of the lodge to allow for entry and egress. The spiritual experience can be enhanced by decorating your sweat lodge with symbolic symbols and materials such as feathers or prayer flags.

•**Construction in Steps**

Constructing your own sweat lodge may be a fun and gratifying experience. While different buildings are employed depending on tribe and cultural traditions, the basic techniques for building a sweat lodge are identical. Here's a step-by-step tutorial for making your own sweat lodge:

Step 1: Gather your Supplies

•**Frame:** You'll need approximately ten to twelve flexible saplings or twigs that can bend without cracking. For this function, red or white cedar, ash, willow, or hazel wood are typically utilized. Plastic can also be used to create a more modern lodge.

•**Covering:** You can cover the frame of the lodge with wool blankets, canvas tarps, or any other form of heavy-duty cloth. Ascertain if the material is non-synthetic and capable of withstanding high temperatures.

•**Roofing:** A huge piece of canvas or tarp will be required to cover the roof of your lodge.

•**Rocks:** To heat in the fire, you'll need roughly 30-40 huge rocks. A free place is required to construct a fire and heat the rocks. For the fire pit, you can use stones, bricks, or metal.

•**Water:** Plenty of water will be required for heating the rocks and drinking during the ceremony.

Step 2: Locate an Appropriate Location

Choose a setting that is private, secluded, and free of distractions or noise.

•**Drainage:** Make sure the place has enough drainage so that water may easily flow away from the sweat lodge.

•**Fire Safety:** Ensure that the environment is fire-safe, with no overhanging trees or flammable materials nearby.

Step 3: Mark the area and excavate a shallow pit.

•**Mark the Sweat Lodge's Circular placement:** Use stones or sticks to mark the sweat lodge's circular placement.

•**Dig a Shallow hole:** Dig a shallow hole in the center of the circle to house the fire and heat the rocks.

Step 4: Build the Frame

•**Form a Dome:** Stick the ends of the saplings or branches into the ground and bend them towards each other to form a dome shape. Make sure the saplings are near enough together to provide a strong structure.

•**Secure the Frame:** Use twine or rope to tie the tops of the saplings together to secure the lodge's frame. If you bind the saplings too tightly, they will snap.

Step 5: Wrap the Frame

•Drape the heavy-duty fabric over the frame and securely wrap it around the framework.

•**Secure with Twine:** Using twine or rope, tie the fabric to the sapling structure. Take caution not to block the sweat lodge's entrance or exit.

Step 6: Light the Fire and Warm the Rocks

•**Build a Fire:** In the shallow pit, start a small fire and gradually add more wood until you have a hot fire going.

•**Heat the Rocks:** Heat the large rocks in the fire until they are red hot. Remove the rocks from the fire with a long-handled shovel.

Step 7: Design the Ceremony

•**Bringing in the Rocks:** Transfer the hot rocks from the fire pit to the center of the sweat lodge with a shovel or tongs.

•Pour water over the hot rocks to create steam, which will fill the sweat lodge with hot, humid air.

•Prayers, singing, and the sharing of spiritual stories are all part of the sweat lodge ceremony. The heat produced by the hot rocks is thought to aid in the purification of the mind, body, and soul.

Step 8: Clean-up

•Allow the hot rocks to cool completely before disposing of them safely in a designated location.

•**Disassemble The Lodge**: After the ceremony, disassemble the frame and carefully dispose of the fabric.

•**Clean up the Area:** Make care to clean up the area thoroughly and leave it as neat as you found it.

Constructing a sweat lodge can be a spiritually fulfilling activity. You may create a safe and functional area for your own sweat lodge ceremony by following these step-by-step instructions and adopting proper safety precautions.

Sweat Lodge Decorations

Keep in mind the spiritual nature of this area and the intention behind each piece you choose to include when you decorate your sweat lodge. Many sweat lodges use natural elements to connect with the earth and create a grounding atmosphere, such as branches, stones, and feathers.

•**Stones:** Because they hold and transmit heat, stones are an essential component of the sweat lodge. Choose polished stones that can resist high heat. Arrange the stones in a circular configuration in the center pit of your sweat lodge to ensure even heat distribution.

•**Prayer ties:** Prayer ties are little bundles tied with string and packed with offerings and intentions, traditionally made of tobacco. To convey intention and connection to your ceremony, hang them from the branches around the sweat lodge.

•**Feathers:** Feathers are frequently used to smudge and cleanse the area before and after the sweat lodge ceremony. They can also be utilized to fan the heated air during the wedding or hanging from the branches.

•**Drumming Instruments**: This can add rhythmic energy to a ritual and help participants connect with one another and the ground. Choose a drum or other instrument that resonates with you and your ceremony's aims.

•**Candles and other light sources:** While the sweat lodge will be dark, consider using candles or other soft light sources to create a peaceful and grounding ambiance.

Remember that your sweat lodge represents an interior journey and a connection to something higher than yourself as you adorn it. Select things and materials that speak to your ceremony's aims and help to create a sacred and meaningful setting for healing and transformation.

Making Use Of Your Sweat Lodge

Respect and preparation are required before using your sweat lodge. The sweat lodge ceremony is usually preceded by a smudging or purification procedure. As a symbol of respect, participants may contribute tobacco, sage, or other sacred medicines to the fire. Once inside the lodge, the leader will lead participants through a number of 15-20 minute rounds. Inside the lodge, stones are brought in and set in the center, where water is poured on them to create steam.

Participants are urged to establish their wishes for the ceremony and connect with the natural environment since this steam is viewed as a physical representation of spiritual energy.

It is critical to remember that the sweat lodge is a sacred location that must be treated with respect. It is also critical to take necessary safety precautions, such as staying hydrated and remaining within one's physical limits. The sweat lodge ceremony allows for spiritual cleansing and connection to oneself and the planet.

CHAPTER 2

NATIVE AMERICAN HERBS

2.1 Horsetail

Horsetail (genus Equisetum), often known as scouring rush, is a genus comprising fifteen species of rushlike visibly joined perennial herbs and the only living plant genus in the order Equisetales and class Equisetopsida. Except for Australasia, horsetails thrive in damp, fertile soils. Some species have two types of shoots: those with cone-like clusters (strobili) of spore capsules and those without. Some are evergreen, while others send up new shoots from underground roots talks every year. Their stems are hollow, jointed, and ridged, and contain silicate and other minerals. The leaves have been whittled down to sheaths that clasp and wrap the sprouts.

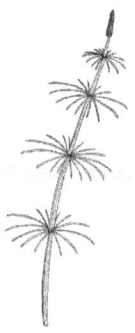

Horsetail

2.2 lemon balm

Lemon balm (Melissa officinalis), sometimes known as balm mild, is a mint family (Lamiaceae) aromatic herb grown for its lemon-scented fragrant leaves. Lemon balm is a Mediterranean and Central Asian native that has naturalized in portions of North America and elsewhere. In temperate climes, it is commonly cultivated as a culinary and medicinal herb, as well as a garden decoration.

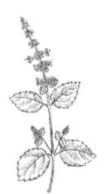

Lemon Balm

2.3 Nettle

Stinging nettle, commonly known as common nettle, is a weedy perennial plant in the nettle family (Urticaceae) with stinging leaves. Stinging nettle is found almost everywhere, but it is most prevalent in Europe, North America, North Africa, and portions of Asia. Young leaves can be cooked and eaten as a healthy potherb, and the plant is commonly used in herbal therapy.

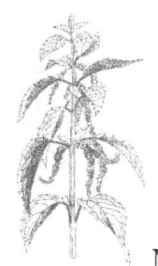

Nettle

2.4 Ginseng:

Ginseng, (genus Panax), Chinese (Wade-Giles romanization) jen sheng or (Pinyin) ren sheng ("root of heaven"), is a genus comprising 12 medicinal herb species in the Araliaceae family. Asian ginseng (Panax ginseng), which is native to Manchuria and Korea, has long been used as a drug and is used to make a stimulating tea in China, Korea, and Japan. American ginseng (P. quinquefolius), which grows from Quebec and Manitoba south to the Gulf of Mexico coasts, is also used in traditional medicine. The majority of produced American ginseng roots are dried and sold to Hong Kong, where the spice is marketed across Southeast Asia.

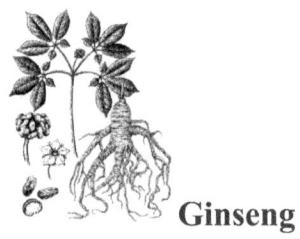 **Ginseng**

2.5 Wild Ginger

Wild ginger, any of approximately 75 species of the genus Asarum, perennial herbs of the birthwort family (Aristolochiaceae) found throughout the world's North Temperate regions. When the leaves and subterranean stems (rhizomes) of some Asarum species are crushed, they emit a pleasant odor, and dried rhizomes are occasionally used as a substitute for ginger.

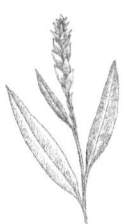

Wild ginger

2.6 Elderberry

Elderberry (genus Sambucus), generally known as elder, is a genus of roughly ten species of shrubs and small trees in the Adoxaceae family. The majority are endemic to temperate or subtropical woody environments in both the Northern and Southern hemispheres. They are valuable as garden shrubs, woodland plants, and for their berries, which feed wildlife and are used to make wines, jellies, pies, and medicines.

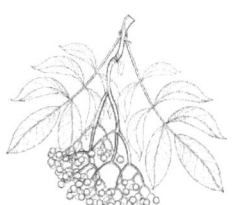

Elderberry

2.7 The Devil's Club

The Devil's club (Oplopanax horridus, Araliaceae; syn. Echinopanax horridus, Fatsia horrida) (Squamish: ch'átyay) (Tlingit: S'áxt) is a big understory shrub native to the Pacific Northwest rainforests, but also found on islands in Lake Superior. It is distinguished by its huge palmate leaves and upright, woody stems that are coated in poisonous and painful spines. It is sometimes known as Alaskan ginseng and other similar names, despite the fact that it is not a true ginseng.

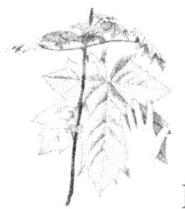

Devil's Club

2.8 Cranberry

Cranberry is any of numerous small creeping or trailing plants in the Vaccinium genus (family Ericaceae), as well as their tart edible red fruits. Cranberries are a popular pie filling in the places where they are cultivated, their juice is widely sold as a beverage, and cranberries in sauce and relish form are traditionally connected with Thanksgiving and Christmas dinners in the United States and Canada.

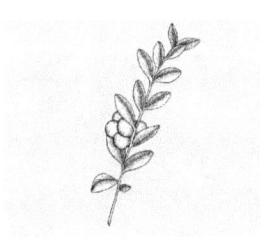

Cranberry

2.9 Chamomile

Usually spelt camomile, any of several daisy-like plants in the asteraceae family. Chamomile tea is produced from English or Roman chamomile (Chamaemelum nobile) or German chamomile (Matricaria chamomilla), and is used as a tonic, antibacterial, and in many herbal treatments.

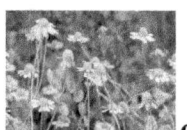chamomile

Several species, particularly golden marguerite and yellow chamomile (Cota tinctoria), are grown as garden ornamentals.

CHAPTER 3

3.1 **Catnip** (Nepeta cataria), often known as catmint, is a mint family (Lamiaceae) herb known for its scented leaves, which are especially appealing to cats. Cat owners frequently plant catnip for their pets, and the dried leaves are frequently used as stuffing for cat toys. The plant is native to Eurasia and is used in some regions as a flavoring as well as a therapeutic tea for colds and fever.

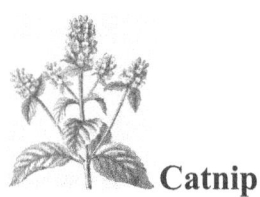
Catnip

3.2 Cattail (genus Typha), genus of approximately 30 species of tall reedy marsh plants (family Typhaceae), primarily found in temperate and frigid regions of the Northern and Southern hemispheres. The plants are aquatic or semi-aquatic and live in fresh to slightly brackish waters. Cattails are beneficial to wildlife, and many varieties are grown ornamentally as pond plants and dried flower arrangements. The large flat leaves of the common cattail (Typha latifolia) are used to make carpets and chair seats in particular. Some people eat the starchy rhizomes.

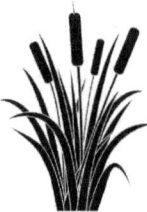

Cattail

3.3 Blueberry :Any of many North American shrubs in the genus Vaccinium (family Ericaceae) are appreciated for their delicious edible fruits. Blueberries, known as a superfood, are high in dietary fiber, vitamin C, vitamin K, manganese, iron, and antioxidants. Blueberries are popular as a dessert fruit and can also be baked into a variety of pastries. Blueberries are linked to cranberries and bilberries, both of which are members of the Vaccinium genus.

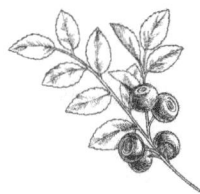

Blueberry

3.4   Lingonberry (Vaccinium vitis-idaea), commonly known as cowberry, foxberry, or rock cranberry, is a tiny creeping plant in the Ericaceae family, related to blueberries and cranberries. Lingonberry plants can be found in boreal woods and tundra locations throughout the Northern Hemisphere. Northern Europeans and Scandinavians in the United States use the red fruit for jelly and juice, while native peoples in North America value it. The plants grow densely and can be collected by raking, just like cranberries.

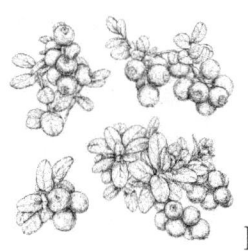

LingonBerry

3.5 Cascara sagrada (Spanish for "sacred bark") is the dried bark of the buckthorn Rhamnus purshiana (order Rosales), which is used as a laxative in medicine. The tree is grown in both North America and Kenya. Cascara sagrada is available in liquid and solid forms. The activity appears to be the consequence of the combined action of numerous compounds, a number of which have been identified and are primarily anthraquinones.

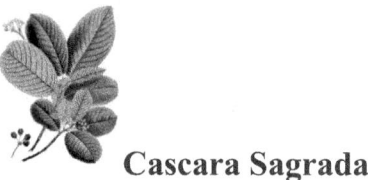 **Cascara Sagrada**

3.6 Boneset (Eupatorium perfoliatum), often known as agueweed, is a plant in the aster family (Asteraceae) native to North America.

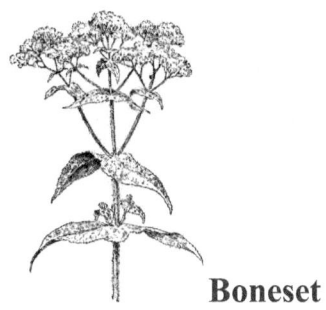

Boneset

The plant attracts butterflies and is sometimes grown in rain gardens. Boneset tea is a folk medicine for fever, and the leaves were historically wrapped around fractured bones to encourage healing.

3.7 Aster (Aster species)
Ojibwa and Pawnee Tribes
Traditional Medicinal Use: Skin irritations
Other: used as a seasoning additive with boiling fish. Medicinally utilized by the Pawnee for skin irritations. The stems were reduced to charcoal before being applied to the skin over the afflicted area. The leaves were used for seasoning by the Ojibwa. The leaves were boiled with fish before being eaten together.

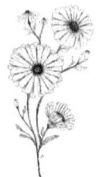

Aster Flower

3.8 Black Eyed Susan (Rudbeckia hirta)

Tribes include the Ojibwa, Menominee, and Potawatomi.

Traditional Medicinal Uses: pediatric assistance, increased urine flow, colds.

The blooms of this plant were utilized as a pediatric aid by the Ojibwa. It was employed by the Menominee for its diuretic effects.

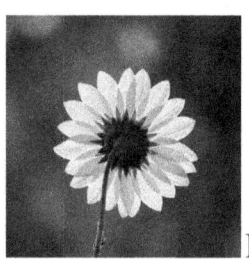**Black Eyed Susan**

3.9 Goldenrod Solidago sp.

Ojibwa and Omaha are two tribes.

Traditional Medical Use : cramping, fever, stomach cramps

Other: This plant serves as a ripening indicator for maize.

In the floral calendar, the Omaha utilized this plant as a mark or indication. When they were on their summer buffalo hunt, they noticed that their maize was starting to ripen back home. For cramping, the Ojibwa brewed a decoction of the root and administered it externally. Fever was treated with a decoction of dried leaves. For stomach cramps, a hot infusion of the root was applied externally.

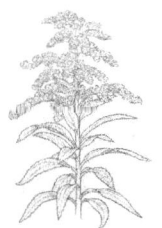

GoldenRod

Goldenrod (genus Solidago), genus of roughly 150 species of weedy, typically perennial asteraceae herbs. The majority of them are native to North

America, with a few species being found in Europe and Asia. Goldenrods are common plants in eastern North America, where there are about 60 kinds. They can be found in practically every habitat type, including woodlands, swamps, mountains, fields, and roadside ditches, and are one of the main floral beauties of autumn from the Great Plains eastward to the Atlantic.

4.0 Physalis virginiana (Prairie Ground Cherry)
Ho Chunk and Dakota tribes
Traditional Medicinal Use: headaches, stomach upset, and wounds
Other activities include eating young greens and playing with children.
The root was utilized by the Ho Chunk to treat headaches and stomach problems. An infusion of the root was used as wound dressing. In the spring, the Dakota ate hard, young, green seed pods with boiling flesh. The children entertained themselves by striking the inflated blooms on the brow or hand.

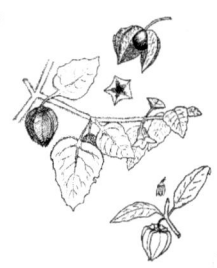

Prairie Ground Cherry

CHAPTER 4

4.1   The herb hyssop (Hyssopus officinalis)

Not specified tribes

Traditional Use: Coughs, fevers, weak stomach, cuts, bruises, asthma, muscular rheumatism, and other lung and chest illnesses are all traditional medicinal uses.

Other: cooking sweetener

Cough syrup, asthma syrup, and other lung and chest disorders were created. Fever was treated with infusions. This plant's leaves were often used to brew tea that was consumed with meals. The tea was brewed with the herb's green tops to improve the tone of a weak stomach. The green tops are also used to treat asthma by boiling them in soup. It was also used in cooking as a sweetening flavor. An infusion of the leaves was used externally to treat muscle rheumatism and bruising.

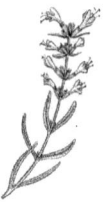

Hyssop

4.2 Marsh Mallow (Althaea Officinalis)
Dakota Indian Tribe
Traditional Medicinal Uses: bruises, sprains, hemorrhages, muscle aches, chest ailments, coughs, bronchitis, whooping cough, inflammation and irritations of the urinary and respiratory organs. The plant's root was largely utilized to make decoctions and thick pastes. A decoction proved beneficial in treating bruises, sprains, and muscle or sinew aches.

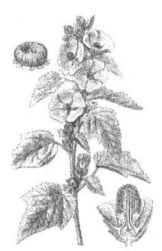

Marshmallow

It has been suggested that the powdered root boiled in milk be used to treat urinary organ hemorrhages and diarrhea. Marsh Mallow, when boiled in wine or milk, was used to treat chest ailments such as coughs, bronchitis, whooping cough, and so on. It was typically combined with other herbal treatments. It was commonly administered in the form of syrup, which was most suited to infants and children.

4.3 Mint (Mentha piperita)
Dakota, Menominee, Omaha, and Pawnee tribes
Traditional Medical Use: Pneumonia, local discomfort, antacid, and gas relief
Other: a beverage, such as tea
Wild mint was utilized as a digestive aid by all nations. It was soaked in water and given to the patient to drink. This infusion was sometimes

consumed as a beverage, similar to tea, not only for its therapeutic properties but also for its pleasant aromatic flavor. For pneumonia, the Menominee prepared a compound infusion and a poultice that was administered to the chest. To ease local pain, crushed fresh leaves were applied.

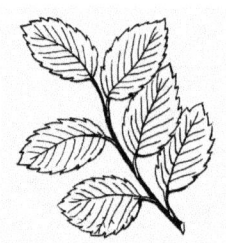

Mint

4.4 Ox Eye Daisy (Leucanthemum vulgare Lam).
Traditional Medicinal Use: fever, night sweats, chronic coughs, bronchial inflammation, pulmonary consumption Tribe: Menominee
Other: honey-sweetened beverage
It operates similarly to Chamomile as a tonic, calming and soothing. It has been suggested as a treatment for night sweats.

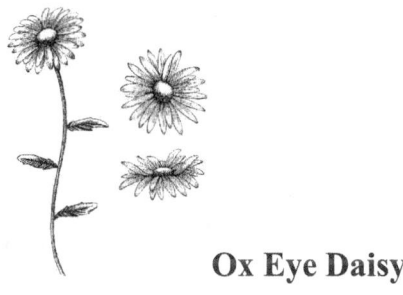

Ox Eye Daisy

The blossoms have a balsamic flavor and make an excellent infusion for treating chronic coughs and bronchial irritation. Boiling the leaves and stalks and sweetening them with honey produces a wonderful drink for the same reason. The root can be consumed through the lungs. This was utilized as a fever remedy by the Menominee.

4.5 Purple Coneflower (Echinacea purpurea) is a type of coneflower.
Dakota and Sioux are two tribes.
Traditional uses include snakebites, stings, burns, toothaches, and toxic conditions.

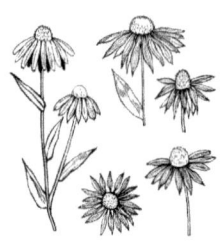

Purple Coneflower

This herb has long been utilized as an antidote for snake bites, stings, and other dangerous situations. It was used in the treatment of headaches with smoking. It was also employed as a toothache treatment, with a portion placed on the affected tooth until relief was obtained. To alleviate pain, burns were washed in the fluids.

4.6 Daucus carota (Queen Anne's Lace)

Not specified tribes

Traditional Use: Colic, liver, kidney, bladder, painful urination, ulcers, abscesses, sores, wounds, enhance menstrual flow, expel worms from the bowels

The petals of Queen Anne's lace were used to make tea; the root and seeds were often pulverized and used for colic, liver, kidney, and bladder problems, painful urination, increasing menstrual flow, and removing worms from the bowels. Grated root poultice was suggested for ulcers, abscesses, sores, and severe wounds.

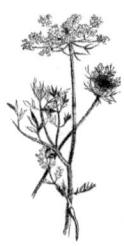

Queen Anne's Lace

4.7 Trifolium pratense (Red Clover)

Tribe : Pawnee

Traditional Medicinal Use: preventive

Other uses: The stiff elastic stems were made into brooms to sweep the lodges.

For a sore and inflamed throat, the leaves were occasionally used to prepare a drink similar to tea. The thick elastic stems were used to build brooms to sweep the lodges, according to the Pawnee. The plant was also utilized to keep diseases at bay.

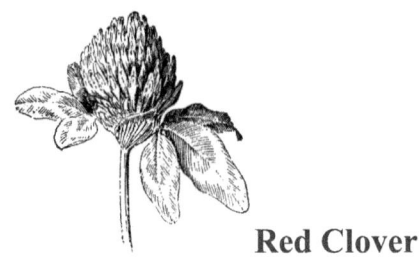

Red Clover

4.8 Wild Strawberry (Fragaria virginiana Duchesne)

Dakota, Ho Chunk, Ojibwa, Omaha, and Pawnee are among the tribes.

Traditional Medicinal Uses: stomach pain, cholera, urine functions

Other examples include fresh fruit and tea prepared from leaves.

Many tribes consumed the berries right off the shrub.Its leaves are very good for tea. This herb was utilized by the Ojibwa to treat cholera and stomach problems.

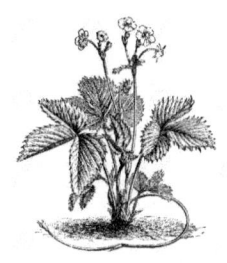 **Wild Strawberry**

4.9 Yarrow (Achillea millefolium)

Tribes include the Ho Chunk, Lakota, Ojibwa, and Potawatomi.

Traditional Use : Swellings, a stimulant, headache, dermatological aid, earache, severe colds, fevers, opens the pores, purifies the blood, measles, other eruptive disorders, suggested in the early stages of children's colds

Other: ceremonial functions

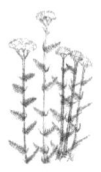 **Yarrow**

The Ho Chunk utilized an infusion of this herb to bathe swellings. A wad of the leaves and the infusion were placed in the ear to relieve earache. Yarrow tea was used to treat severe colds, fevers, and cases of blocked sweating. It readily opens the pores and purifies the blood. It was advised to use it in the early stages of a child's cold, measles, and other eruptive disorders. The Ojibwa burned flowers and utilized the smoke to treat fevers. Flowers were sometimes burned for ceremonial purposes. For headaches, a decoction of leaves was cooked and inhaled. For dermatological purposes, the root was applied to the skin. A dried root was chewed and spit upon the limbs as a stimulant.

HERBAL BIBLE BOOK 4

CHAPTER 1: HERBS

1.1 Coneflower (Rudbeckia laciniata L.)
Ojibwa Tribe
Traditional Medicinal Use: burns, indigestion
The Ojibwa used a flower compound poultice to treat burns. Indigestion was treated with a compound infusion of the root.

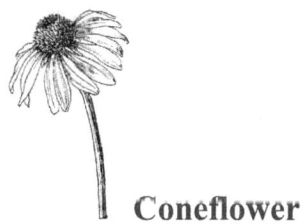

Coneflower

1.2 Wood Sorrel (Oxalis acetosella)
Tribe : Menominee, Omaha, and Pawnee tribes
Traditional Medicinal Uses: cooling agent, high fever, relieve thirst, mouth ulcers, heal wounds, stop

bleeding, cure or prevent scurvy, stimulate urine output, reduce swellings and inflammation
Other ingredients: yellow dye

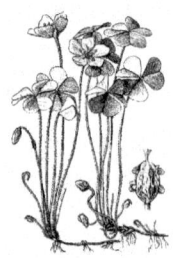

Wood Sorrel

For high fevers, a beverage produced from its pleasant acid leaves was given to quench thirst as well as to alleviate the fever. The juice of the leaves was concentrated into a fine, clear syrup that was as effective as an infusion. The juice was used as a gargle to treat mouth ulcers, as well as to cure wounds and stop bleeding. Sponges and linen cloths soaked in the juice and applied to the body were thought to be useful in reducing swellings and irritation. The Menominee used the entire plant as a yellow dye after boiling it.

1.3 Agave:

Agave (genus Agave), one of the 200 species of the Asparagaceae (previously Agavaceae) family, is native to the Americas' dry and semiarid regions, mainly Mexico and the Caribbean. The genus has a variety of economically significant species, particularly those necessary for the manufacturing of mescal liquors, such as blue agave (Agave tequilana), which is used to make tequila. Sisal (A. sisalana), henequen (A. fourcroydes), and cantala (A. cantala) are high-fiber plants with potential as bioenergy crops. The principal sources of agave nectar, a syrupy sweetener, are the century plant, or maguey (A. americana), and blue agave. A variety of species are also grown as ornamentals in desert landscaping.

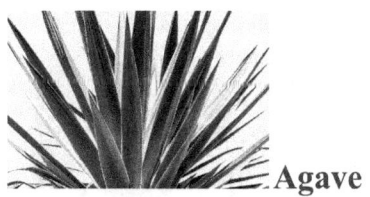
Agave

1.4 Oregon grape: any of several species of the genus Mahonia, evergreen shrubs of the barberry family (Berberidaceae) used for decorative

purposes. M. aquifolium, the common Oregon grape, grows to be 90 cm (3 feet) tall and is native to North America's Pacific coast. It is mainly famous for its foliage, which consists of glossy, leathery leaves with five to nine leaflets that are spiny-edged like holly. Small yellow fragrant blooms in terminal clusters are followed by small blue edible berries that can be turned into jelly.

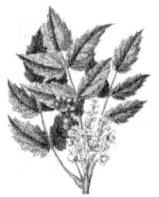

Oregon grape

1.5 Pine, (genus Pinus), genus comprising approximately 115 species of evergreen conifers of the pine family (Pinaceae), spread globally but predominantly endemic to northern temperate climates. Pines and other conifers are important members of the world's taiga (boreal forests), coniferous forests, and mixed forests, and many pine species are iconic or characteristic constituents of a number of specific ecosystems, such as the southern United States' longleaf pine (Pinus palustris) ecosystem.

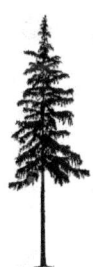

pine

The plants, like other trees, provide habitat and a range of other ecosystem services, and pine seeds are an essential source of food for birds, squirrels, and other animals. Pines have the highest economic importance in the construction and paper industries, but they are also a source of turpentine, rosin, oils, and wood tars. Several species produce edible pine seeds, which are sold commercially as pine nuts, pignoli, pions, or pinyons. Many pines, including black, white, Himalayan, and stone pines, are grown as ornamentals, and some are used in reforestation programmes or as windbreaks. Pine-leaf oil, which is used medicinally, is a distillation byproduct of the leaves; distillation byproducts include charcoal, lampblack, and fuel gasses.

1.6 Yucca (genus Yucca), genus of roughly 40 species of succulent plants endemic to southern North America in the agave subfamily of the asparagus family (Asparagaceae). The majority of yucca species are stemless, with a rosette of stiff sword-shaped leaves and clusters of waxy white blooms at the base.

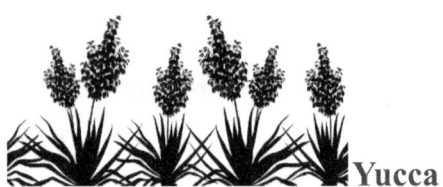
Yucca

1.7 The spider plant

Members of the genus are perennial evergreen plants that grow to be little taller than 60 cm (2 feet). The roots are fleshy and tuberous, and rhizomes (underground stems) are used by numerous species to spread. Typically, the long, narrow leaves are positioned basally. Small bisexual flowers are produced on a thin floral spike, and some species develop clonal plantlets that root easily to produce new plants.

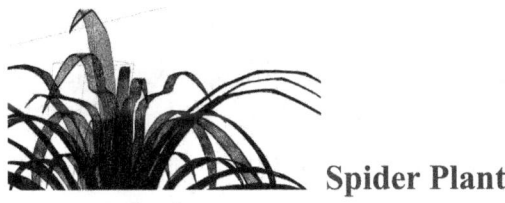

Spider Plant

1.8   Purslane, any of a number of tiny, fleshy annual plants in the genus Portulaca (40-100 species), family Portulacaceae. The plants feature protruding, generally reddish stems, spoon-shaped leaves, and flowers that open in the sun.

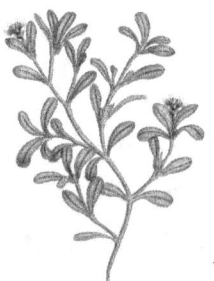

Purslane

The common purslane (P. oleracea), sometimes known as pusley, is a common weed distinguished by its little yellow blooms. P. oleracea sativa, often known as kitchen garden pusley, is produced as a potherb, primarily in Europe. Rose moss (P. grandiflora), a trailing fleshy plant with vividly coloured, sometimes doubled flowers, is grown as a garden decoration. All plants in the genus are notable for their tenacity; they can grow well even in dry waste soil and hold enough moisture to bloom and ripen seeds even after being removed. The capsules, which open with a lid, disperse numerous little seeds of exceptional longevity.

1.9 Peppermint (Mentha piperita) is a fragrant perennial herb in the mint family (Lamiaceae). Peppermint has a strong sweetish odor, a warm pungent flavor, and a cooling aftertaste. Fresh leaves are used as a culinary herb, and dried blooms are used to flavor candies, pastries, beverages, salads, and other meals. Its essential oil is also commonly used to flavor foods. The plant, which is a cross between watermint (Mentha aquatica) and spearmint (Mentha spicata), is grown throughout Europe, Asia, and North America.

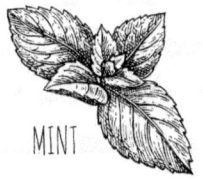

MINT

2.0 Evening primrose is a type of primrose.
The common evening-primrose, Oenothera biennis, is a flowering plant in the Onagraceae family that is native to eastern and central North America, from Newfoundland west to Alberta, southeast to Florida, and southwest to Texas, and has become widely naturalized elsewhere in temperate and subtropical regions.The plant is used to make evening primrose oil.

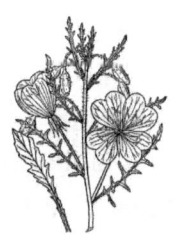

Evening primrose

CHAPTER 2: NATIVE HERBS

2.1 Prickly ash (genus Zanthoxylum), genus of approximately 200 aromatic trees and shrubs of the rue family (Rutaceae) endemic to the intermediate latitudes of North America, South America, Africa, Asia, and Australia.

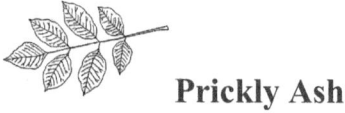 **Prickly Ash**

Several species are grown as ornamentals or for their beautiful wood, and others are utilized in herbal medicine. Sichuan pepper, an Asian spice, is made from the dried husks of many species' fruits, including Zanthoxylum piperitum, Z. simulans, and Z. bungeanum. Prickly ash is another name for the unrelated angelica tree, often known as devil's walkingstick (Aralia spinosa).

2.2 Amaranth (genus Amaranthus), genus containing 60-70 species of flowering plants in the Amaranthaceae family, found almost everywhere. Several amaranth species are grown for their leaves as well as for edible seeds, which are a nutritious pseudocereal (non grass seeds utilized like cereal grains). Amaranthus caudatus, prince's feather (Amaranthus hypochondriacus), and Joseph's coat (Amaranthus tricolor) are all common garden ornamentals. Several species are classified as weeds.

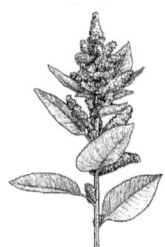

Amaranth

2.3 Sage (Salvia officinalis), often known as common sage or garden sage, is an aromatic herb of the mint family (Lamiaceae) grown for its pungent edible leaves. Sage is a Mediterranean native that is used as a seasoning in a variety of cuisines, particularly stuffings for poultry and pig and sausages. Some types are planted as ornamentals because of their beautiful leaves and blossoms. Several other Salvia species are also referred to as sage.

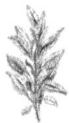

Sage

2.4 Clover (genus Trifolium) is a genus of around 300 annual and perennial species in the pea family (Fabaceae). Clovers are found in most temperate and subtropical regions of the world, with the exception of Southeast Asia and Australia; cultivated forms have naturalized in temperate locations around the world. The plants can be utilized as livestock feed, sown as a cover crop, or used as green manure. The blossoms are very appealing to bees, and clover honey is a common byproduct of clover farming.

Clover

2.5 Witch hazel, any of five species of Hamamelis (family Hamamelidaceae), all of which are shrubs and small trees native to eastern North America and eastern Asia. Some are planted for their yellow flowers, which have four short, twisted ribbonlike petals and bloom during the winter or early spring. Witch hazels have deciduous, strongly veined, oval, toothed leaves and produce little clusters of four-petaled flowers close to the branches.

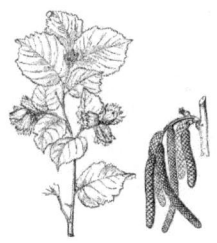

Witch Hazel

2.6 Hawthorn, commonly known as thornapple, is a wide genus of thorny shrubs or small trees in the rose family (Rosaceae) belonging to the northern temperate zone. Many species are native to North America, while other cultivated forms are planted as ornamentals due to their lovely flowers and fruits. The hawthorn is also useful for making hedges, and its mix of tough twigs, firm wood, and numerous thorns makes it a formidable barrier to livestock and wildlife.

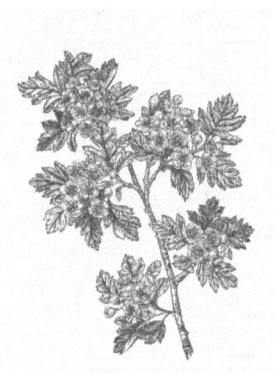

Hawthorn

2.7 Aloe vera is a succulent plant species in the Aloe genus.It is widely dispersed and considered an invasive species in many parts of the world.It is an evergreen perennial that originated in the Arabian Peninsula but now grows in tropical, semi-tropical, and dry conditions all over the world.It is grown for commercial purposes, mostly as a topical therapy that has been used for centuries.The species is appealing as an ornamental plant and thrives inside as a potted plant.

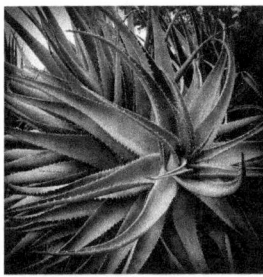**Aloevera**

Aloe vera leaves contain considerable amounts of the polysaccharide gel acemannan, which can be utilized topically.Aloe skin contains the poisonous aloin. Typically, Aloe vera products just employ the gel.

2.8 Blackberry lily (Iris domestica), often known as leopard lily, is a beautiful garden flower and a perennial flowering plant of the iris family

(Iridaceae). It is native to East Asia and has become naturalized in portions of North America. The plant, despite its name, is not a genuine lily; it was previously known as Belamcanda chinensis.

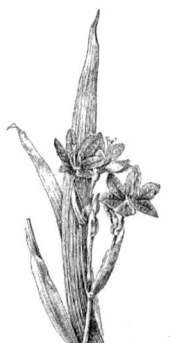

Blackberry Lily

2.9 Barberry, any of the over 500 species of thorny evergreen or deciduous shrubs in the genus Berberis of the Berberidaceae family, predominantly native to the North Temperate Zone, particularly Asia. Species of Oregon grape, once classified as Berberis but now classified as Mahonia, are commonly referred to as barberry.

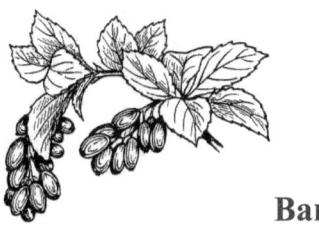

Barberry

3.0 Wormwood, any of several bitter or aromatic herbs or shrubs of the genus Artemisia of the aster family (Asteraceae) found across the world. Several wormwood species are grown for their essential oils, which are used as flavorings or in herbal medicine. The plants feature several little greenish yellow flower heads that are arranged in clusters. The leaves are typically split and alternating along the stem; they might be green, grayish green, or silvery white in color.

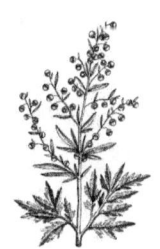

Wormwood

CHAPTER 3: HERBS

3.1 Valerian (Valeriana officinalis, Caprifoliaceae) is a European and Asian perennial flowering plant.In the summer, when the mature plant can reach a height of 1.5 meters (5 feet), it produces delightfully scented pink or white blooms that attract a variety of insect species, particularly hoverflies of the genus Eristalis.

Some Lepidoptera (butterfly and moth) larvae, like the gray pug, eat it as food.Although crude extract of valerian root may have sedative and anxiolytic effects and is often offered as dietary supplement capsules to induce sleep, clinical evidence that it is beneficial for this purpose is currently poor or unclear.Its roots and leaves elicit a catnip-like reaction in cats.

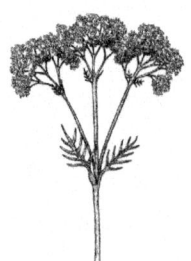

Valerian

3.2 English yew (Taxus baccata), sometimes known as common yew or European yew (all three are lumber trade names), is a beautiful evergreen tree or shrub in the Taxaceae family that grows throughout Europe and Asia as far east as the Himalayas. Some botanists regard the Himalayan variety as a distinct species, Himalayan yew (Taxus wallichiana).

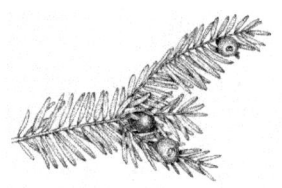

Yew

The tree grows to a height of 10 to 30 meters (35 to 100 feet), with spreading branches and gently drooping branchlets. The bark is reddish brown and flaky, with deep fissures in older trees. Yews are one of the few conifers that can easily sprout new growth from the tips of cut branches; as a result,

English yew is one of the only conifers that is frequently trimmed into hedges. Except for the fleshy aril around the seed, all portions of the English yew contain alkaloids that are toxic to humans and several other species. Thrushes and other birds have been observed digesting the aril and passing the seed intact in their droppings after consuming the seed whole.

3.3 Saint-John's-wort (genus Hypericum), genus comprising roughly 500 species of temperate and tropical herbs or low shrubs in the Hypericaceae family. Several species are grown for their beautiful flowers, and at least one, common Saint-John's-wort (Hypericum perforatum), is used in herbalism. The common name comes from the fact that several European varieties bloom around June 24, which is St. John the Baptist's feast day; "wort" comes from an Old English term for herb or plant.The genus's members have simple opposite or whorled leaves that are gland-dotted and usually have smooth margins. The flowers are typically yellow with five petals. They are distinguished by a profusion of stamens, which are frequently arranged in bundles. The fruits are almost invariably dry capsules.

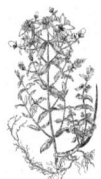

Saint John's wort

The common, or perforated, Saint-John's-wort (H. perforatum), which is native to Europe, Northern Africa, and Western Asia, is one of the most well-known species. The plant is used in herbal therapy to treat depression, and there is some limited clinical evidence that it works. It is toxic to grazing animals, causing photosensitization, behavioral disorders, sudden abortion, and death. The plant spreads asexually via creeping rhizomes and quickly reseeds itself with seeds that can survive in the soil seed bank for years. In southern Australia, South Africa, and North and South America, it has become a noxious invasive species. Certain beetle species (Chrysolina quadrigemina, C. hyperici, and Agrilus hyperici) have been introduced in many regions in the western United States, where it is often known as Klamath weed, to devour the plants and keep them under control.

3.4 Anise (Pimpinella anisum), annual herb of the parsley family (Apiaceae), farmed mostly for its aniseed fruits, the flavor of which is similar to that of licorice. Anise, which originated in Egypt and the eastern Mediterranean region, is now grown throughout southern Europe, southern Russia, the Middle East, North Africa, Pakistan, China, Chile, Mexico, and the United States.An unrelated plant with a similar flavor profile is star anise.

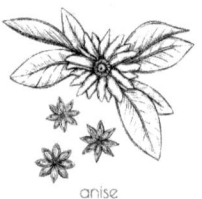

Anise

3.5 Angelica (genus Angelica), genus comprising roughly 90 aromatic herbs of the Apiaceae family native to the Northern Hemisphere. Several varieties are edible and have long been used in herbal medicine, particularly in China. Because the plants resemble deadly species such as poison hemlock

(Conium maculatum), water hemlock (Cicuta species), and hogweed (Heracleum species), they should not be consumed until their identity is known.

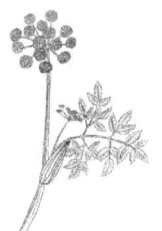

Angelica

3.6 Watercress (Nasturtium officinale), sometimes known as cress, is a perennial aquatic plant of the mustard family (Brassicaceae) that is native to Eurasia and has become naturalized throughout North America. Watercress grows submerged, floating on the water, or scattered on mud surfaces in cool flowing streams. It is frequently grown in tanks or moist soil for its tasty young shoots and delicate peppery-flavored leaves that are high in vitamin C.

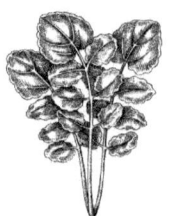

WaterCress

The decorative nasturtium (genus Tropaeolum) is not related to watercress.Watercress plants grow in dense colonies and root freely from their stems. The pinnately compound alternating leaves have three to nine leaflets. Each seedpod, known as a silique, contains two rows of seeds and bears compact clusters of small four-petaled white flowers.

3.7 Goldenseal, also known as Orangeroot or Yellow Puccoon, is a perennial herb native to the forests of the eastern United States. Its rootstocks are therapeutic in nature. The plant produces a single greenish white flower with falling petals, followed by a cluster of little red berries. Goldenseal is occasionally planted in the shaded wild garden, but it is also farmed commercially for the yellow rootstocks that produce hydrastine, an alkaloid.This and a related Japanese species belong to the

Hydrastidae family, while other authorities classify them as Ranunculaceae (buttercups).

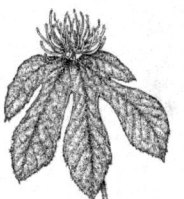

Goldenseal

3.8 Black cohosh often known as black bugbane, black snakeroot, rattle-top, or fairy candle (syn. Cimicifuga racemosa), is a flowering plant in the Ranunculaceae family. Its range extends from the extreme south of Ontario through central Georgia, and west to Missouri and Arkansas. It thrives in a wide range of woodland settings, but is most commonly seen in small woodland openings. Native Americans employed the roots and rhizomes in traditional medicine. Its extracts are used to make herbal medications or dietary supplements.

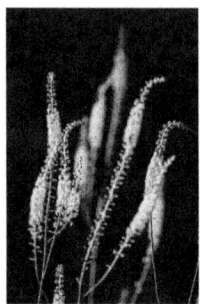 **Black Cohosh**

Most dietary supplements containing black cohosh have not been well researched or approved for safe and effective treatment of menopausal symptoms or any disease.Some herbal medicinal products containing black cohosh extract, on the other hand, have a marketing authorization in several European Union states and are well-studied and recommended for safe and effective use in the relief of menopausal symptoms (i.e. in the years surrounding menopause) such as hot flushes and profuse sweating attacks.This distinction between product types appears to be significant.

3.9 Sassafras, also known as Ague Tree, is a North American tree of the laurel family (Lauraceae) whose aromatic leaf, bark, and root are used as a flavoring, traditional home medicine, and tea. The roots generate about 2% sassafras oil, which was historically a key ingredient in root beer.From Maine through Ontario and Iowa, and south to Florida and Texas, the tree is endemic to sandy soils. It is normally modest, but can grow to be 20 m (65 feet) tall or more. It has furrowed bark, bright green twigs, and little clusters of yellow flowers that bloom before producing dark blue berries. Sassafras has three types of leaves, which are often seen on the same twig: three-lobed, two-lobed (or mitten-shaped), and entire.

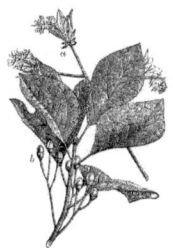

Sassafras

4.0 The Slippery Elm: orred elm, and large-leaved elm (Ulmus rubra or U. fulva) of eastern North America have strong wood and fragrant inner bark. The inner bark contains a glue-like material that has long been soaked in water as a treatment for throat illnesses, powdered for use in poultices, and chewed as a thirst quencher, among other things. It has recently earned fresh attention as part of alternative medicine's herbal pharmacopeia, being given for a wide range of diseases.

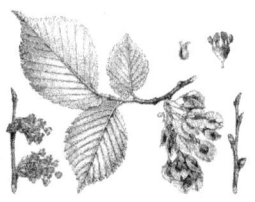

Slippery Elm

4.1 Bloodroot (Sanguinaria canadensis), often known as red puccoon, is a poppy (Papaveraceae) plant native to eastern and midwestern North America. It grows in deciduous woodlands and flowers in early spring; it is occasionally cultivated as an ornamental. Native Americans used to color using the orange-red sap of the rhizomes. The rhizomes also contain the alkaloid sanguinarine, which is used in medicine.

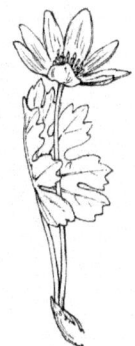

BloodRoot

Despite the fact that the plant is toxic, overharvesting for use as a herbal medicine and unproven cancer treatment has decimated wild populations across much of its native habitat.Bloodroot has a cup-shaped flower with eight petals and vivid yellow stamens (male reproductive organs) in the middle. A 20-cm reddish stem supports the 4- to 6-cm (2-inch) bloom. The flower stem is encased in a big veiny half-opened leaf. The leaf unfolds into a multi-lobed blue-green spherical form after the flower blooms. To attract ants for dissemination, the seeds have fleshy structures called elaiosomes.

4.2 Passion flower (genus Passiflora), usually spelt passionflower, is a genus of around 500 species of primarily tendril-bearing vines in the Passifloraceae family and their distinctive flowers. The majority of species are located in the Americas' neotropical regions. Some are grown for their decorative value, while others are grown for their delicious fruits. Many are significant butterfly larval host plants.

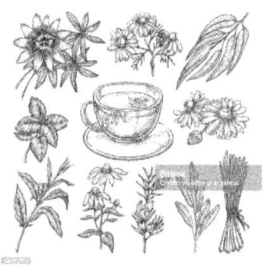

Passion Flower

HERBAL BIBLE   BOOK 5

CHAPTER 1: HOME MADE HERBAL SOLUTIONS FOR DISEASES

1.1   ASTHMA   AND   ITS   HERBAL REMEDIES

Also known as bronchial asthma.

A condition in which a person's airways become inflamed, constrict, swell, and create excess mucus, making breathing difficult.

Asthma can be mild or severe, interfering with daily activities. It may result in a life-threatening attack in some situations.

Herbal Treatments arc listed below

Asthma tea:

Ginger includes chemicals known as gingerols and shogaols, which may provide brief relief from asthma symptoms.

Green tea is high in antioxidants, which may help reduce inflammation associated with asthma. It contains caffeine, which may temporarily relax your airways.

Caffeine, found in black tea, is a stimulant that may enhance lung function and provide brief relief from asthma symptoms.

Licorice tea is prepared from licorice root extract, which may help reduce asthma symptoms when taken with other treatments.

Mullein may alleviate asthma symptoms by relaxing respiratory muscles. Remember that further human studies are required.

1.2 BACKACHE AND ITS HERBAL REMEDIES

Back ache/pain is a physical discomfort that happens at the lower back and this ranges from slight to acute on the spine specifically.

Common Reasons:

Back discomfort might have causes other than an underlying disease. Overuse can include excessive exercise or lifting, extended sitting and lying down, sleeping in an uncomfortable position or wearing a poorly fitted rucksack.

Herbal Treatments are listed below

1. Devil's Claw Tea
Devil's claw is a well-known herb for back discomfort. This intriguingly named South African herb is high in anti-inflammatory chemicals known as iridoid glycosides. Devil's claw, in particular, contains harpagoside, a natural pain reliever.

2. Willow Branches
Willow bark was the inspiration for aspirin because it contains salicin, which transforms to salicylic acid, the main active element in aspirin.
As a result, willow bark is frequently utilised as a herbal headache cure. However, it is also useful against other types of pain, including lower back pain.

3. Curcumin

Turmeric is frequently prescribed for muscle and joint discomfort since its major active element, curcumin, is an anti-inflammatory. According to laboratory research, the curcumin in turmeric can reduce inflammation in the cells of our spinal discs, which may help to alleviate back pain.

4 . Piperine

Piperine is a herb with powerful anti-inflammatory effects that is found in black pepper. It has already showed promise in the treatment of sciatica, and its capacity to relieve inflammation may also help with other types of back pain.

Another advantage of piperine is that it promotes the absorption of curcumin, so it's common to advocate taking these two herbs together.

5 . Green Tea

Green tea provides numerous advantages due to high quantities of antioxidants and anti-inflammatory substances like EGCG. One way it helps with back pain is by preserving our bodies' cartilage from injury and degeneration. This can help to prevent back discomfort as well as joint pain.

6 . Ginger .

Ginger is another excellent anti-inflammatory plant. This flaming root is a natural pain reliever that can help with persistent lower back pain, muscle discomfort, and joint pain, among other things. Ginger can also be used to relieve tense neck muscles.

1.3 ALLERGIES , RASHES AND ITS HERBAL REMEDIES

Skin Rash is also known as Cutaneous condition.
A brief outbreak of red, rough, scaly, or itchy patches of skin, possibly accompanied by blisters or welts.

Common Reasons:

Skin rashes can have reasons other than an underlying disease. Hot and humid temperatures, excessive sun exposure, or scratchy garments that don't fit are all examples.

You may be wondering what a red, swollen, itchy, and painful patch on your skin is. It could be a rash. A rash can be an indication of a number of medical issues. It can be caused by an irritant (a substance that causes irritation) or allergies. Because a rash can be caused by a variety of factors, determining the actual cause is critical in order to receive effective therapy.

Certain substances may cause you to develop a rash if they come into contact with your skin. As a result, rashes can also be caused by skin allergies. Even though a rash is unpleasant and painful, it is not communicable. It cannot, therefore, pass from one person to another.

However, there are several home cures for skin rashes that you may find effective in soothing your skin. But, before we get there, there are a few things we should be aware of.

Skin allergies and rashes are widespread since we come into contact with a variety of potential allergens during our daily activities. Your herbal doctor will advise you on the best course of treatment for these rashes. Even after starting treatment, the rash may take some time to disappear.

If you are looking for natural remedies for rashes and skin allergies, you might consider home remedies for skin rashes.

Herbal Treatments are listed below

1. Chamomile

Matricaria recutita L. is the scientific name for German chamomile. Externally, the flower can be used to treat skin inflammation, rashes, and eczema, as well as many other allergic skin problems. Human studies demonstrate that it is more effective in the treatment of skin allergies and rashes .

As a home cure for skin allergies, make a tea with a few tablespoons of German chamomile leaves and consume it. It is also a component of several ointments on the market. You can also apply the German chamomile flower extract to the rash by forming a paste of the flowers and gently dabbing it on it.

2. Sage Leaves

One of the home cures for skin rashes is sage leaf. Sage is a Mediterranean medicinal plant that has long been used in herbal medicine to treat mild skin inflammations. Certain chemicals contained in sage were proven to have anti-inflammatory activities in laboratory and animal investigations.

It is not suggested for use in children under the age of 18, as well as pregnant or lactating mothers. As an at-home skin rash treatment, apply sage oil prepared from the sage leaf gently over the rash with a cotton swab.

3 . Evening Primrose

Evening primrose was found to decrease the symptoms of atopic dermatitis in a clinical investigation. It was also discovered to alleviate eczema symptoms when applied topically to rashes. As a result, you can use evening primrose as a home treatment for skin allergies. It may aid in the reduction of skin irritation, dryness, itch, and exfoliation (the elimination of dead cells).

Please keep in mind that it should not be used by anyone suffering from schizophrenia or epilepsy, children, or pregnant or breastfeeding women. By combining a few drops of evening primrose essential oil in tea and drinking it, you can use it as a natural home cure for skin rashes. You can also use the essential oil to treat rashes.

1.4   SORE THROAT AND IT HERBAL REMEDIES

Sore throat is also known as Pharyngitis.
Pain or irritation in the throat, which can occur with or without swallowing, is frequently associated with diseases such as the common cold or flu.

Common Reasons

A sore throat can have causes other than an underlying ailment. Overuse of the voice, a burn from hot food, an extremely dry mouth, or sleeping with the mouth open are all examples.

Herbal Treatments are listed below

1. Cinnamon

Warming cinnamon is a lovely spice to add to your herbal tea to make it extra soothing, especially if your throat is sore. Cinnamon is antimicrobial by nature, making it an excellent choice for combating throat infections and colds.

Cinnamon is also a natural analgesic. It is also high in antioxidants, making it a powerful anti-inflammatory agent.

2. Tea With Slippery Elm

For millennia, slippery elm has been used as a natural medicine.It mixed with water it forms a gel-like material and that's because it contains mucilage. When you drink slippery elm tea, the gel can coat your throat, soothing and protecting it when it is irritated.

4. Tea with Chamomile

Chamomile tea has long been used for therapeutic purposes, including healing sore throats. It is anti-inflammatory, anti-oxidant, and astringent.

CHAPTER 2

2.1 CRAMPS AND IT'S HERBAL REMEDIES

Cramp is a painful, uncontrollable muscular contraction that's experienced by female gender.

Common Reasons

Cramps can have reasons other than an underlying condition. Dehydration, severe exercise, and a lack of muscular use are a few examples.

Painful period cramps, often known as dysmenorrhea, affect approximately 50% of women. You don't have to suffer through this pain; natural therapies such as diet, herbs, and certain nutrients can help reduce or eliminate the discomfort you feel during "that time of the month."

Herbal Treatment are listed below

1.Ginger : is my number one choice for cramp relief. One study found that taking ginger capsules four times a day for three days before your period works just as well as ibuprofen for treating menstrual discomfort. I've noticed some significant reductions in cramping pain after using this warming herb. Ginger is also useful for nausea, so I like to prescribe it to ladies who have cramping discomfort along with nausea, vomiting, and bloating at the start of their period. Aside from ginger capsules, you can incorporate more ginger into your diet throughout the month. Here are some ways to add ginger into your diet:

•Consume freshly pressed juice including ginger, lemon, cucumber, and other greens.

•Make fresh ginger tea: Bring to a boil, then cover and simmer sliced fresh ginger root for 15 minutes, then add sliced lemon for another 5-10 minutes, sweeten with honey, and drink daily.

•In the morning, add a thumb-sized piece of fresh ginger to your smoothies.

•In a pinch, replace your second cup of coffee with ginger tea bags.

•Make a warming turmeric tea latte with fresh ginger root (at least 2 tsp).

2.2 ACNE AND IT'S HERBAL REMEDIES

Acne is a common skin Disease that results in the breakout of pimples. Acne commonly appears on your face. Acne is caused by clogged pores.Among teenagers and young adults and also adults Acne occurs. There are herbal treatments available to clear your skin ,avoid scars and make it smooth.

Herbal Treatment are listed below

1.Witch Hazel

Witch hazel contains astringent tannins that may help treat acne by eliminating excess skin oil. It's also anti-inflammatory and can help with redness and bruising. Witch hazel is frequently used on its own or as a base for Do-it-yourself acne treatments.

2.Tea Tree

Tea tree (melaleuca alternifolia) is a plant that is used to heal skin conditions and wounds. Its antibacterial and anti-inflammatory properties may help to minimize the amount of acne lesions. In a 1990 study, a topical gel containing 5% tea tree oil was compared to a topical cream containing 5% benzoyl peroxide. Both treatments reduced the amount of acne lesions, both inflamed and noninflamed. Although tea tree oil took longer to function, it had less adverse effects. Dryness, itching, inflammation, and redness were among them.

Other antibacterial and anti-inflammatory herbs that may aid in acne healing include:

Calendula, chamomile, lavender, and rosemary are all herbs.

2.3   ANEMIA   AND   IT'S   HERBAL   REMEDIES

Anemia is a condition that's caused by lack of sufficient red blood cells that are healthy in the blood. Anemia is caused by a shortage of or malfunction of red blood cells in the body. This results in decreased oxygen supply to the body's organs.

Herbal Treatment are listed below

1.Dandelion

There are two possible reasons for iron deficiency anemia: not consuming enough iron-rich foods or not absorbing it effectively. In any event, dandelions has your back. Its leaves not only have significant levels of iron, but they also help the body absorb this crucial element. This plant can be combined with others to increase its effectiveness, as in this Anti-Anemia Dandelion and Nettle Tea.

2.Nettle

This herb, often known as stinging nettle, is abundant in iron. However, the presence of vitamins A (retinol), B group, C (ascorbic acid), and K, all of which promote iron absorption in the body, makes it even more helpful. Nettle consumption for anemia recovery is not only healthy, but also simple. It can be used as a tonic, tea, or supplement, or it can be used in the same manner as iron-rich spinach is to make pesto sauce and salads.

3. Parsley

Parsley, a prominent green herb native to the Mediterranean region, is extremely beneficial in the treatment of anemia. This is due to the high percentage of iron it contains. People who have difficulty swallowing iron supplements are frequently advised to consume parsley juice or tea. Parsley is far more than simply a garnish; it is a strong medicinal plant for those suffering from anemia. Amaranth, soy sprouts, and quinoa are other excellent sources of iron.

HERBAL BIBLE BOOK 6

CHAPTER 1

1.1 STRESS AND ITS HERBAL REMEDIES

A state of worry or mental tension generated by a challenging situation is defined as stress. Stress is a natural human response that motivates us to deal with problems and risks in our lives. To some extent, everyone is stressed.

Herbal Treatment are listed below

1.Lavender

Lavender is a popular herb due to its lovely perfume and enticing flavor. But did you know it also has considerable anti-anxiety and anti-depressant properties? It has long been used to offer relaxation and aid in the treatment of anxiety and PTSD (post-traumatic stress disorder).In aromatherapy, essential oil of lavender is mostly used. It helps to lower cortisol levels in the body, which helps to control anxiety symptoms. Lavender leaves can also be used to produce an aromatic and calming cup of tea.

2. Passiflora incarnata (passionflower)

Passionflower is a well-known herb that helps to treat depression and anxiety, as well as uneasiness and insomnia. It is also indicated for anxiety relief and relaxation. Some specialists believe it is also beneficial for those experiencing menopausal symptoms including hot flashes.

3. Matricaria recutita (chamomile)

Chamomile is a herb that has been used as a natural cure for anxiety and agitation for millennia. You can ingest it in the form of tea (the most frequent), pills, or extracts. Chamomile includes phenolics that aid to relieve stress, such as flavonoids, quinones, phenolic acids, and antioxidant molecules. It can also be used to alleviate menstrual cramps, relieve tension, and promote relaxation.

1.2 FIBROID AND ITS HERBAL REMEDIES

Fibroid is also known as uterine myoma. Non Cancerous uterine growths that can occur throughout a woman's reproductive years.

The exact cause of fibroids is unknown. A family history of fibroids, obesity, or the onset of puberty at a young age are all risk factors.

Herbal Treatments are listed below

1.Green tea

Green tea includes antioxidant compounds known as flavonoids.Antioxidants help in the prevention of cell damage in the human body by reducing oxidative stress. Oxidative stress is a major cause of disease.

2. Curcumin

Curcumin is one of the Important active compounds in turmeric. It is antibacterial, anti-inflammatory, and antioxidant.

According to certain studies, Trusted Source curcumin can destroy fibrotic cells or prevent them from replicating. Again, cell cultures are the foundation of these investigations, and researchers must examine its effects on humans to see whether it will be effective.

1.3 COLD,COUGH AND IT'S HERBAL REMEDIES

The common cold is caused by a viral infection of the upper respiratory tract. A rhinovirus is the most common cause, and the most typical symptoms include a stuffy or runny nose, sneezing, and a scratchy, sore throat.

The common cold's first symptoms are very obvious: a stuffy or runny nose, sneezing, and a scratchy, sore throat. Because the common cold is so widespread, most individuals readily recognise these early symptoms. Adults, on average, get 2 to 3 colds every year.

Herbal Treatments are listed below

Some herbs are naturally effective at treating cold and flu symptoms like coughs, sore throats, and congestion. In truth, many diverse cultures around the world have used catnip, cayenne, echinacea, garlic, ginger, peppermint, rosemary, thyme, and yarrow for millennia.

1.Catnip

Catnip promotes sleep, improves digestion, reduces stomach discomfort, stimulates hunger, and has antibacterial effects.

Origins Catnip was used as a therapeutic herb as early as 1735, when the use of catnip leaves and blossoms in herbal teas was mentioned in the General Irish Herbal.

What to do with it: To create tea, use 1-2 tablespoons of catnip per cup of water. Pour boiling water over the catnip in a tea infuser. Allow the mixture to steep for 15-20 minutes, covered.

2.Cayenne Pepper

Cayenne pepper is used to improve circulation, increase appetite, aid digestion, boost energy, clear sinuses, cause skin-cooling sweats in hot weather, and warm up in cold weather. It can also be applied topically as a counter irritant, bringing blood to the skin's surface and relieving arthritis.

Origins: Cayenne Pepper originated in Cayenne, the capital of French Guiana, and is called for the city. It was first planted around 7,000 years ago in Mexico and over 4,000 years ago in Peru. In the 1400s, Christopher Columbus introduced it to Europe. It is now cultivated in India, East Africa, Mexico, and the United States.

What to do with it: Because cayenne can cause heartburn in some people, it should be added to the diet a pinch at a time. Cayenne pepper can be put with tomato juice to reduce cold symptoms if you're used to it and don't have digestive issues. Use 14 to 12 teaspoon dry cayenne pepper per pint tomato juice. Only consume 12 to 1 cup at a time and store the rest in the refrigerator.

3. Echinacea

Echinacea is often used to treat infections caused by viruses and bacteria, to increase immunity.

Origins: Despite being one of the most well-known and commonly used therapeutic herbs on the list, Echinacea has a relatively brief history of use. Its roots can be traced back to the indigenous Indian nations of North America. The earliest archaeological evidence was discovered in the 18th century.

What to do with it: Typically, the root of echinacea is used to make ointments, tonics, or teas, although the aerial section of the plant has also been utilized successfully in some formulations. Because the active components in echinacea aren't water-soluble, making a tincture is the best method to gain its advantages.

Ingredients

• 34 cup 80-100 proof vodka

• A quarter cup of distilled water

• 12 oz. chopped echinacea root

Directions

• In a jar with a tight-fitting cover, combine the alcohol and water.

• Echinacea root is optional.

• Release trapped air bubbles along the jar's edge using a knife or chopstick.

• Put the lid on the jar and store it in a cold, dark area for 2 weeks.

• Every day, shake the mixture.

• Remove the chopped root and strain the mixture into another jar with a tight-fitting lid. Replace the cover immediately to prevent the alcohol from evaporating.

•Label the tincture and keep it in a cool, dark place. It has a 5-year shelf life.

•Take 30 drops of the tincture every 3 hours for two days at the first indication of a cold or flu.

4. Garlic

Garlic has antibacterial, antiviral, and antiparasitic properties. It also has several cardiovascular benefits, such as lowering blood cholesterol and blood pressure.

Origins: Garlic is one of the most anciently known cultivated herbs. According to certain sources, garlic was produced in China as long as 4000 years ago. Garlic has been used by numerous societies throughout history, despite the fact that it only grows wild in Central Asia. The Egyptians believed it improved strength and endurance while also preventing disease. Greek athletes consumed it prior to competition, and Greek warriors consumed it prior to battle. It was also reported that Roman troops carried it into combat.

What to do with it: Garlic is best used by eating it or crushing or chopping cloves into foods. To reap the benefits of its therapeutic characteristics, take two cloves every day.

5. Ginger

Ginger is well known for its digestive system effects, including its ability to reduce nausea and indigestion, stimulate the digestive tract, and aid in digestion. It can, however, be used topically as a counter-irritant, increasing circulation and alleviating cold and flu symptoms by clearing sinuses and generating perspiration for fevers.

Origins: Ginger was first employed in ancient Chinese cultures and expanded over the Indo-Pacific and India as early as 3050 B.C. It was one of the first Asian spices to be exported.

What to do with it: Ginger can be found in teas and other liquids that support digestive health or soothe upset stomachs. However, it can also be used fresh, like garlic, for similar relief. Add a tablespoon to your favorite stir fry or grate some ginger root into a salad to reap the benefits.

CHAPTER 2

2.1 CONSTIPATION AND ITS HERBAL REMEDIES

Constipation is a difficulty passing feces. Constipation is defined as passing less than three stools per week or having difficulty passing stool.

Constipation is a pretty frequent condition. Constipation can be caused by a lack of dietary fiber, water, and exercise. However, other medical conditions or medications may be at blame.

Constipation is a healthy challenge that makes one have not less than three bowel movements, hard stool and always very difficult to pass and sometimes lumpy stool. You can normally take actions to avoid or relieve constipation.

Herbal Treatments are listed below

1.Buckthorn (Cascara sagrada)

This is a popular herbal laxative derived from the bark of a buckthorn tree species. This substance stimulates bowel motions by irritating the colon. Although short-term use is generally well tolerated, it may produce gastrointestinal pain or electrolyte imbalance. Long-term use can result in liver damage ranging from mild to severe.

2. Psyllium

Psyllium, a plantain plant species, is a natural fiber laxative that aids in the formation of bulky stools. Psyllium is frequently used to treat persistent constipation and can be coupled with various natural and synthetic laxatives.

3. Elm Slippery

This herb has a long history of being used to treat constipation. It stimulates nerves in the gastrointestinal (GI) tract, causing mucus production and relieving constipation. There has been little investigation into the long-term implications. Mucilage, a sticky material found in slippery elm, covers the GI tract. As a result, if used concurrently, it may impair the absorption of several drugs.

4. Peppermint : is used to treat a number of stomach problems. It alleviates gas and stomach cramping, stimulates bile production to facilitate digestion, and reduces nausea and vomiting. When eaten, it can also cause perspiration and clamminess, as well as promote alertness. It can be applied topically to ease pain, relax muscles, and relieve itching and achy muscles. Peppermint also has antibacterial qualities.

Origins: In the late 1600s, peppermint was first cultivated in England. It has, however, been used to cure indigestion since 1000 B.C. in ancient Egypt. Peppermint is a natural hybrid of spearmint and watermint that has been utilized by Egyptians, Greeks, Romans, early Christians, Mediaeval Europeans, and North American colonists throughout history.

What to do with it: Peppermint tea is commonly used to alleviate stomach issues. For 10-20 minutes, steep 1 tablespoon fresh chopped peppermint or 1 teaspoon dried peppermint in 1 cup hot water. While the tea steeps, keep it covered.

2.2   INSOMNIA AND ITS HERBAL REMEDIES

Insomnia is the Consistent difficulty of falling and staying asleep. The majority of cases of insomnia are caused by poor sleeping habits, sadness, anxiety, a lack of exercise, a chronic ailment, or a specific prescription.

Herbal Treatments are listed below

1.Lavender

Lavender is a well-known herb for promoting sleep and relaxation. The majority of studies on the effect of lavender on sleep have focused on silexan, an active ingredient produced from lavender.

2. Chamomile

Is occasionally used as a natural treatment for insomnia. However, investigations on the therapeutic effects of chamomile on sleep have not been conclusive.

3. Saint John's Wort
is a weed that thrives in pastures. In truth, their development must be regulated since they can be lethal to grazing cattle, but because they have certain therapeutic properties, they are often referred to as weedy herbs. This weed, yellow blossoms are high in tryptophan, which promotes serotonin synthesis.

Serotonin alleviates depressive symptoms, setting the way for a restful night's sleep. The plant makes the skin become so receptive to natural light. Avoid exposing your skin to direct sunlight immediately after applying this herb-infused oil to your skin.

2.3   WRINKLES AND IT'S HERBAL REMEDIES

Skin aging is inevitable; your skin will alter over time and you will notice it. Your skin has wrinkles and fine lines. Chemical treatment is a quick option, but it's still a chemical, so shooting chemicals into your face doesn't sound pleasant and isn't cheap either. So here are some herbs that can help your skin and reduce the effects of aging. Here's a list of them.

Herbal Treatments are listed below

1.Basil

Holy basil, also known as tulsi, aids in the prevention of aging. Excessive UV exposure causes skin damage and collagen loss. Soak the basil leaves in warm water for 10 minutes to soften and form a paste. Apply it to your face after mixing it with graham flour and honey. Once dried.

2.Ginger

Ginger contains a high concentration of antioxidants and anti-inflammatory compounds, which aid in the prevention of aging. Grated ginger, brown sugar, and olive oil are required. Apply it all together for 10 minutes, then wash it off.

3. Ginseng

This Chinese medicinal herb is well-known for its anti-aging properties. Mix a teaspoon of ginseng powder with a cup of warm water and apply it on your face using a cotton ball. The safest method is to leave it overnight.

4. Horsetail

It contains natural silicon, which can help you achieve youthful, beautiful skin. You will need chopped horsetail shoots and honey. After two days, drain the honey and ingest the plant. For best effects, consume it twice daily.

2.4. SUNBURN AND IT'S HERBAL REMEDIES

A form of skin burn caused by overexposure to sunshine or sunlamps. Repeated exposure raises the chance of developing other problems like wrinkles, dark patches, and skin cancer.

But, let's face it, sunburns happen, and even with the best of intentions and attempts, there will always be the unintentional nap on the beach or the strange burn from propping your elbow along the open car window. Fortunately, relaxing relief is closer than you think. Here are five essential herbs to keep on hand for sunburn recovery (together with instructions on how to use them in a salve or tonic):

1.Basil
Although basil is commonly used in cooking, it has a long history of medical applications. The herb can relieve sunburn that is still at the ouch-ouch stage

2. Calendula
Calendula is a charmer and one of the most commonly used medicinal herbs throughout history. The plant not only has beautiful yellow-and-orange blossoms, but it's also a terrific addition to natural beauty treatments.

3. Oregano
Oregano was a favorite of Hippocrates, and it is still used as a remedy for sore throats in Greece. This plant, like basil, is ideal when you start to feel

tender. It's an excellent addition to any anti-sunburn pack.

4. Rosemary
Another culinary favorite, rosemary, can provide antioxidants to the skin, which can only help your sunburn treatment.

You should make a salve with basil, calendula, oregano, and/or rosemary. Here's how to go about it:

•To begin, make an infused oil by combining dried or fresh plant pieces in a glass jar with olive oil.

•Then, a few weeks before your beach day, set the jar in a warm, sunny window (the sunlight helps to break down the plant pieces).

•Shake the jar at least once a day, and then drain the mixture and bottle it in a new container when ready to use.

•Use the oil directly on your skin, or combine it with coconut oil or an unscented moisturizer to make the base for a salve.

5. Valerian

If a sunburn is bothering you enough to keep you awake at night, try valerian, the ultimate sleep aid. Traditionally used as a herbal sedative, you can create a tea from the dried roots or prepare a "tonic wine" by steeping around two ounces of the dried root in a cup of dry white wine for at least a few days.

SYNOPSIS AND CONCLUSION

The" Indigenous American Herbal Bible: 6 in 1 Book of Ancestral Medicinal Plants with images" by Joseph F. Peraza is a thorough guide that delves into Native American civilizations' rich and old herbal traditions. This six-in-one foraging book encapsulates the information, wisdom, and practices passed down through centuries, offering a unique perspective on the world of indigenous medicine.

The book opens by emphasizing the significance of comprehending the natural environment, which serves as the foundation for Native American herbalism. It introduces readers to a wide range of medicinal plants, each with its own unique set of uses and healing capabilities. For millennia, these herbs have played an important part in Native American cultures' health and well-being, and Peraza's work ensures that this knowledge is kept and disseminated.

The emphasis on sustainability and ethical foraging is one of the book's most fascinating components. It emphasizes the need of respecting nature and its resources, which is consistent with Native American beliefs about the interdependence of all living things. This speaks to modern readers who are looking for more sustainable and holistic approaches to health and wellness.

As we conclude, "Indigenous American Herbal Bible" provides a link between traditional knowledge and modern herbalism. It instills a deep reverence for the environment while also providing practical insights into the usage of native plants for healing and wellness. For people interested in herbal medicine, traditional knowledge, and the preservation of Native American heritage, Joseph F. Peraza's work is an important resource. It provides as a thorough guide to the many practises of indigenous herbalism with its six-in-one approach, making it an essential addition to the library of anybody interested in the healing potential of plants and a deeper connection to the natural world.